INSIGHTs on Nutrition & Weight Loss

A Guide to Losing Weight and Keeping It Off

Jason Conviser, Ph.D., FACSM

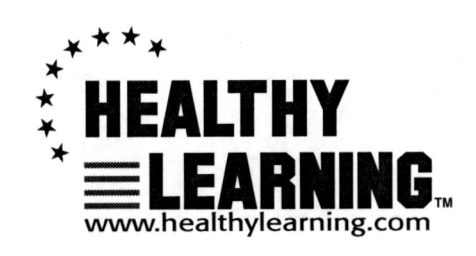

HEALTHY LEARNING
www.healthylearning.com

©2012 Healthy Learning. All rights reserved. Printed in the United States.

No part of this book may be reproduced, stored in a retrieval system, or transmitted, in any form or by any means, electronic, mechanical, photocopying, recording, or otherwise, without the prior permission of Healthy Learning. Throughout this book, the masculine shall be deemed to include the feminine and vice versa.

Chapters 1-2 and 10-11 are adapted with permission from Bookspan (2008). *Health & Fitness in Plain English: How to Be Healthy, Happy, and Fit for the Rest of Your Life* (Third Edition). Monterey, CA: Healthy Learning.

Chapter 1, Chapters 3-9, and the Glossary are adapted with permission from Kruskall (2010). *Fitness Professionals' Guide to Sports Nutrition and Weight Management*. Monterey, CA: Healthy Learning.

Chapter 12 is adapted with permission from Ratamess (2006). *Coaches' Guide to Performance-Enhancing Supplements*. Monterey, CA: Coaches Choice.

Chapter 13 is adapted with permission from Benardot & Thompson (2007). *The Coaches' Guide to Sports Nutrition*. Monterey, CA: Coaches Choice.

ISBN: 978-1-60679-223-0
Library of Congress Control Number: 2012938524
Cover design: Roger W. Rybkowski
Book layout: Roger W. Rybkowski
Front cover photos (clockwise from top): Hemera/Thinkstock; Noel Hendrickson; iStockphoto/Thinkstock; Courtesy of NuStep

Healthy Learning
P.O. Box 1828
Monterey, CA 93942
www.healthylearning.com

Dedication

I first met Mark Stephan in August of 2008, six months after he suffered a catastrophic head and spine injury as a result of a cycling accident. Few thought that he would survive, and doctors told his family that Mark was destined for a life confined to a wheelchair. Less than four years later, I am in San Diego, California, with Mark as he prepares to be the first "functional" quadriplegic to ride a specially designed tricycle across America, in an effort to raise awareness for athletes who have overcome great challenges in their life, as well as to raise money for the Rehabilitation Institute of Chicago. I dedicate this book to Mark and to all athletes who have overcome great physical challenges. Mark, I wish you great success over the next 3,129 miles and commit all of my royalties from the sale of this book to the Stephan Challenge and Rehabilitation Institute of Chicago.

Jason Conviser
April 15, 2012

In Memory

Seldom, if ever, does an individual have the opportunity to recognize publicly someone who was special throughout their life. Two years ago, Aubrey Greenberg passed away after a short illness. Aubrey was more than just an uncle to me—throughout my life, he was a mentor, guide, critic, fishing partner, supporter of my dreams, warrior on my behalf, and friend. Many of the "things" that I have accomplished today are because of him. Everyone should be so lucky as to have someone like Aubrey in their life! Aubrey Greenberg may no longer be present in my life on a daily basis, but he has not been forgotten.

Acknowledgments

It's a rare and wonderful opportunity to be able to recognize and thank those who have helped me in so many ways throughout the years and especially in development of this manuscript. Thanks go to Dr. James Peterson, publisher of Healthy Learning/Coaches Choice, for his continued support in my career. Thank you to Kristi Huelsing for her many editorial hours with this manuscript and design of the final product. Thank you to Dr. Bill Ciganek for his keen medical knowledge and ability to extract fact from fiction within the scientific literature. There have been many people who have given their time, writing, and insights into this book on nutrition and weight loss, helping to ensure it focuses on the intended audience without going over their heads with facts they will never use. Thanks to Drs. Bookspan, Kruskall, Ratamess, Benardot, and Thompson for their great work. Thanks to Dr. James S. Skinner for his friendship and for partnering with me in lectures throughout the world. Thank you to James Freedman for his counsel and for sharing wonderful family adventures each year and to Lauren Freedman for her support and friendship for over 30 years. Thank you to clients whom I also consider my friends—I have learned so much from JK, CG, RJ, RM, TP, MS, KB, MK, JL, and RW. My love to Rebecca, Sarah, and Nathan, three of the most important parts of my life—you are exceeding every dream I ever had for each of you. You make a father very proud. Finally, I would like to thank Dr. Jenny Conviser, my wife, who has been a great supporter and, when needed, critic. She is one of the industry leaders in weight management, eating disorders, and behavioral psychology, but is also my best friend.

Contents

Dedication 3
Acknowledgments 4
Preface 7

Section 1: That Makes Sense—Why Didn't I Think About That Before? 9
Chapter 1: Half Truths, Almost Lies, and Things Marketers Will Claim
to Entice You to Purchase Their Products 11
Chapter 2: Healthy Weight-Management Habits 33

Section 2: Exercise Nutrition—What You Need To Know 49
Chapter 3: Carbohydrates 51
Chapter 4: Lipids 65
Chapter 5: Proteins 71
Chapter 6: Vitamins and Minerals 81
Chapter 7: Hydration—Everything You Need to Know About
Fluids and Electrolytes 87

Section 3: Energy Balance and Weight Management 93
Chapter 8: Energy Balance 95
Chapter 9: Weight-Loss Principles 99

Section 4: Sport Performance Nutrition 113
Chapter 10: Sport Drinks 115
Chapter 11: Performance-Enhancing Foods 121
Chapter 12: Sport Supplement Basics 141
Chapter 13: Getting to the Right Weight and Body Composition
for Athletic Success 153

Section 5: Glossary 163

About the Author 173

Preface

Americans spend more than $40 billion per year on weight-loss products and yet each and every year we hear stories of Americans getting heavier and heavier. The statistics are daunting. For many individuals, losing weight and keeping it off is, at best, a difficult undertaking. From a scientific perspective, the key to weight loss is to achieve a negative caloric energy balance. In other words, individuals need to burn (utilize) more calories than they consume. Sounds simple, and yet our clients tell us over and over again they are overwhelmed with conflicting "information" in newspapers, in magazines, and on television by self-acclaimed experts—all telling them what to do for proper nutrition and how to lose weight.

In fact, losing weight effectively and efficiently involves more than simply eating less. Not only do people need to expend more calories through a more physically active lifestyle, they need to be aware of how what they eat affects their energy equation. They also need to be patient. If it took them more than four weeks to put on those extra pounds, they shouldn't expect to lose them in four weeks or less. Statistics show that an estimated 66 percent of American adults and nearly 20 percent of American children and adolescents are either overweight or obese. As such, much remains to be done in the effort to attain a meaningful and manageable weight loss.

What makes the equation even more difficult is that a single plan does not seem to work for everyone. What is right for an athlete may not be right for a grandmother. What is required by a high school teenager may not be the same as an office worker or an individual who needs to lose a significant amount of weight. Although no one perfect plan exists, there is a way that everyone can become more knowledgeable about nutrition and the scientific principles of sound weight management.

Featuring cutting-edge information on sound weight management, this book was written to provide individuals who want to win the weight-loss battle with a tool that will enable them to be successful. From weight control principles to myths and misunderstandings about losing weight, this book is designed as a must-have resource for anyone who wants to safely lose weight and keep it off.

J.C.

Notice

The information on nutrition and weight management presented in this book is intended to be a guideline, rather than an absolute standard of care for each and every person. In reality, the body of knowledge concerning nutrition and weight management is ever-changing. As new research and clinical experience broaden this knowledge, changes in programming and standards are required. The authors and the publisher have checked with sources believed to be reliable in their efforts to provide information that is complete and in accord with the standards accepted at the time of publication. However, in view of the possibility of human error or changes in industry standards, neither the authors nor the publisher nor any other party who has been involved in the preparation or publication of this work warrants that the information contained herein is in every respect complete, and they are not responsible for any errors or omissions or the results obtained from the use of such information. Readers are encouraged to confirm the information contained herein with their physician with regard to the application of this information to their health and general well-being.

Section One

That Makes Sense— Why Didn't I Think About That Before?

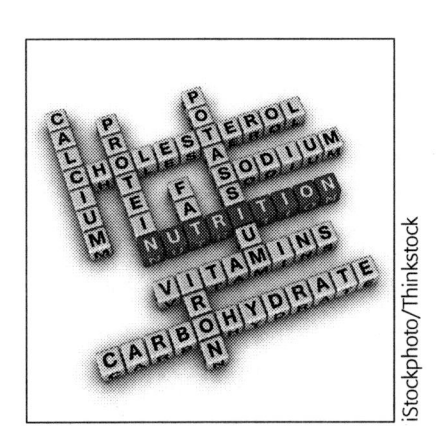

CHAPTER 1
HALF TRUTHS, ALMOST LIES,
AND THINGS MARKETERS WILL CLAIM TO ENTICE YOU TO PURCHASE THEIR PRODUCTS

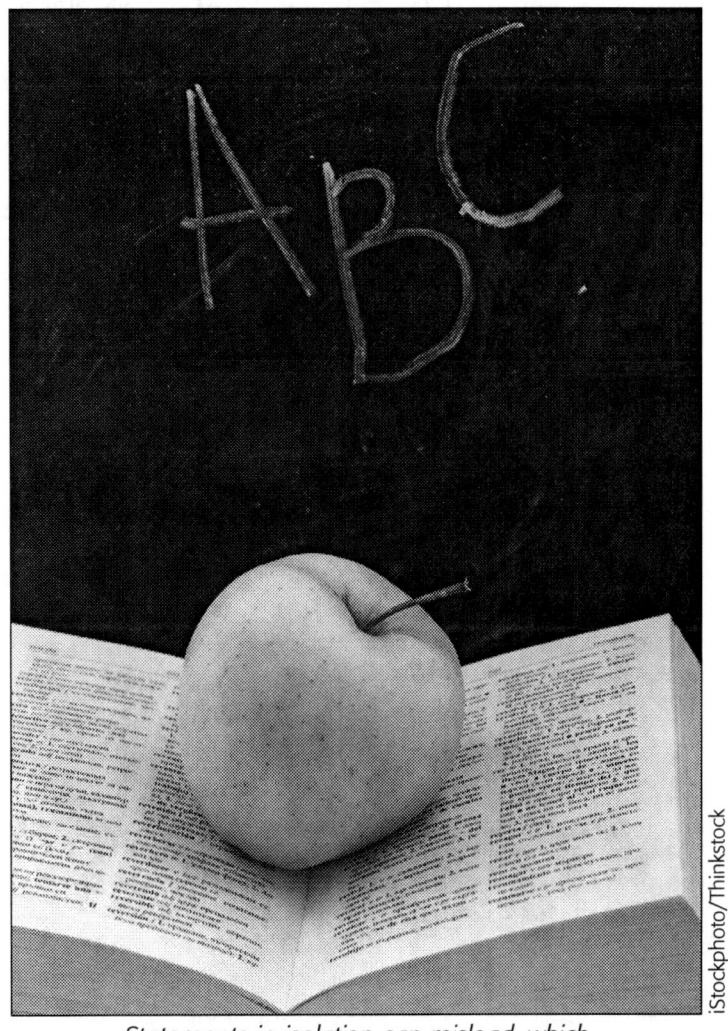

Statements in isolation can mislead, which is how many nutrition myths begin.

If you heard of a nutrient that your body requires to transmit nervous-system signals and manufacture sex hormones and that is a precursor of the bile that handles ingested fats, would you want lots of it in your bloodstream? It's cholesterol.

Would you pay a lot for a substance your brain can't do without to process decisions and retain memory? It's sugar.

Do you avoid a common practice using a chemical that constricts brain blood vessels, reducing cerebral blood flow? It's breathing oxygen.

Nutrition Myths

Statements in isolation can mislead, which is how many nutrition myths begin. Ordinary food items become income producers to the slick packager. Nutrition myths are no exception. Recognizing these myths is part of being an insightful consumer.

The "Isolated Aspect" Myth

Oxygen, in high concentrations, is toxic to every life form on the planet. If you breathe high levels for long periods, you will suffer ill effects. Yet, you don't avoid breathing oxygen in the air around you. You use it for other characteristics in its favor, like staying alive. In similar ways, vitamin and food-supplement advertisements divert your focus to and from isolated aspects of their product. They concentrate on problems occurring only from excesses or deficiencies, or on only one effect of the substance, usually exaggerated.

Claims
- A powdered muscle-building supplement for athletes and people wishing to bodybuild advertises that it is insulinogenic. The suffix *-gen* comes from a Greek word meaning "producing." In other words, it encourages insulin production. The advertising states that insulin is instrumental in getting the building blocks of protein into your muscle cells, and since this product is insulinogenic, it therefore builds muscle. Wouldn't that be great?
- Another product uses the opposite property of insulin for marketing. A popular high-protein diet promotes the idea that you must avoid non-protein foods because they stimulate insulin. Since another property of insulin is to promote fat storage, these people say to eat only high-protein, non-insulin-stimulating foods, to be in a fat-burning "zone."

Critical Reading
- Insulin has several functions. It stimulates the uptake of amino acids into your cells for protein synthesis. It also activates enzymes, which stimulate fat cells to synthesize and store fat. That process is part of how you digest food. The function

of insulin to store fat is left out of advertising for insulinogenic muscle-building supplements. They tell you only about storing protein. The function of insulin to help store protein is left out of promotions for fad diets that limit carbohydrate.
- Two opposite, seriously unhealthful practices are centered around isolated beliefs about insulin. Certain bodybuilders illegally inject insulin, trying to build muscle and create a look of thinner skin because they believe insulin will build muscle. At the same time, a growing subpopulation of people with insulin-dependent diabetes skip or reduce prescribed injected amounts, believing it will reduce body fat, a practice popularly called "diabulemia."
- Almost all food is insulinogenic. Every time food enters the non-diabetic bloodstream, it stimulates insulin release. Nothing is particularly special about a specific "insulinogenic" muscle-building product. It's just food.
- Claims for high-protein diets are misleading and potentially unhealthy. High-protein diets (and other diets) "work" to produce weight loss when they are low-calorie, not because of any insulin-stimulating or suppressing quality.
- Some diets are centered around the insulin-producing quality of food. They rate foods according to their ability to raise blood sugar, called the glycemic index. They avoid high-index foods and stress lower index foods. It is an important and healthful practice to limit junk fat and sugar and eating too much of any food that raises blood sugar and insulin levels frequently. In a few cases, helpful foods are restricted for having a high index, such as carrots, while milk products produce high insulin responses even with a low glycemic index. In general, it is unhealthy to have high and continual insulin responses from constant eating of any food, particularly junk fat and sugar. Use common sense and healthful control to eat smaller portions of more healthful food. Don't rely on artificial products or unhealthful practices, or get bogged down counting numbers and grams and zones. Eat with moderation. Relax.

The "More the Merrier" Myth

Most of your brain is water. Almost no one would expect to get more brain tissue by drinking more water. If you eat an extra portion of something, your body doesn't always necessarily use it to do what you hope it will do. The most flagrant examples involve protein and calcium supplements.

By themselves, protein and calcium won't grow muscles or strengthen bones. Your body continually "turns over" the protein in muscle fibers, calcium in bone cells, and fat in fat cells. It uses some for body function, recycles some, and takes small amounts of incoming material from food for rebuilding. The constant breakdown and resynthesis is called modeling. Modeling doesn't grab extra protein or calcium and add it on to you. It takes what it needs to keep you the same as before and discards the rest, unless you give your body a reason to make you different than before. That reason is resistance exercise, which includes weight lifting and pushing and pulling against resistance. Resistance exercise will make your body add more protein to your muscles, and calcium to your bones. By itself, eating a food will not.

Given normal functions of vitamins in your body, a common assumption is that taking more vitamins must do more of that process. The B vitamins, for example, work as coenzymes. Coenzymes help an enzyme do its enzyme job. The enzyme/coenzyme interdependence is like a lock-and-key relationship. Only one key fits one companion lock. Taking more of a vitamin when your body is not making more of the corresponding enzyme will have no effect; from three wheels you can still make only one bicycle. Taking the companion enzyme in pill form will not help because eating the pills destroys the enzymes, as described in the "No Digestion" myth.

A precursor of bile, a fluid that handles fat digestion, is cholesterol. However, if you eat more cholesterol, your body will still not digest more fat. Your body uses what cholesterol it needs and dumps the rest back into circulation. Too much cholesterol can create unhealthy effects.

The "More Can't Hurt" Myth

Claim
- Protein builds muscles; therefore, more protein must build more muscle, and after all, more can't hurt.

Critical Reading
- Extra protein doesn't build extra muscle unless plenty of resistance exercise tells your body that the muscle is needed.
- Even then, your body can use only so much, regardless of how much you exercise.
- Past that amount, extra protein can be harmful.

Problems of Too Much Protein

Extra protein is not stored; it goes several routes. One is through your excretory system, taking water with it to produce urea. With excessive protein intake, you can dehydrate yourself a bit. Another exit route for excess protein is conversion to fat, which can't be turned back to protein later. Another problem with too much protein is that it increases calcium loss through the urine. In other words, eating too much protein makes you "pee" out calcium. Epidemiologic studies point to excess protein, particularly animal protein, as contributing to osteoporosis.

What about high-protein diets that claim you need extra protein to get you into a fat-burning zone? It turns out that if you follow their meal plans, the meals are low calorie, and for that reason, you lose weight. It does not have anything to do with extra protein, or insulin, or zones. Problems occur because the meals are also low-complex carbohydrate, meaning decreased intake of important nutritional components needed for health. You need energy to carry out daily activities, and to exercise for weight loss and health.

Problems of Too Much Iron

A high blood-iron level is also frequently thought to be a good thing. It is not always true. Iron is essential to your health in several roles. Iron is also involved in certain harmful reactions in your body, involving special molecules called free radicals. Free radicals can sometimes be destructive in your body, which is their job. People with high iron levels have been found to develop high rates of heart disease, possibly from high amounts of free radicals generated through too much iron.

Although women are frequently labeled as at a disadvantage for tendency to lower iron levels than men, it seems that may be an advantage. Populations with lower-than-average iron levels have been found to have lower-than-average incidence of heart disease. Iron supplements are also constipating. It is now a common recommendation that people should not supplement iron without physician recommendation.

Problems of Too Much Water

Even drinking water can be overdone. Extreme prolonged exercise in the heat with no food or fluid replacement other than large amounts of water, or drinking extreme quantities of plain water, for example in a hazing ritual, can cause a problem called water intoxication. Seizures, even deaths, have resulted from an imbalance of the sodium, potassium, and water levels in the body.

More is not always better. Philosopher Allen Ross Anderson encapsulated maximalist thinking: "We should have our minds open, but not so open that our brains fall out."

The "No Digestion" Myth

More is not always better. Sometimes, more becomes nothing at all. Some health food stores sell pills containing enzymes. The claims are that your body needs these enzymes for various functions, so if you eat a supply of these enzymes in their pills, you will get more of the benefits. This claim does not work.

Enzymes do not pass into your bloodstream after eating them. They cannot pass through your intestinal wall except by breaking down into constituent parts. This process destroys them as enzymes.

Broken-down enzymes will not automatically reassemble on the other side of your intestine, so eating enzymes will not raise your body levels of enzymes. Your body makes all the enzymes you need out of the ordinary food you eat. Eating enzymes by themselves, except those that aid digestion (like lactase to digest dairy products), is useless and expensive.

An interesting example is superoxide dismutase (SOD). SOD is an enzyme. It is one of several antioxidants your body makes to counter effects of free radicals. Free radicals have an unpaired electron, so they go around trying to get another electron by taking one from other molecules in your body. Free radicals particularly target fatty acids and proteins, harming them in the process of stealing their electrons. Then, the fatty acids and proteins become free radicals themselves, and go around grabbing electrons from other molecules, like a destructive game of tag. Your body has several built-in systems for removing radicals, but can get overwhelmed by too many free radicals, which can then go unchecked in their damage.

Eating SOD in pill form won't protect against free-radical damage or other oxidative stress in your body. If eaten, SOD, like any other enzyme, is destroyed in your intestine by digestion.

As is often the case with sham cures offered in pill form, research studies seem to back up the claims. Studies do show that SOD reduces free-radical formation. None of these studies involved eating the SOD, but injecting it into laboratory animals under specific conditions. More on free radicals, oxygen toxicity, and antioxidants can be found in the "Reverse Reasoning" myth.

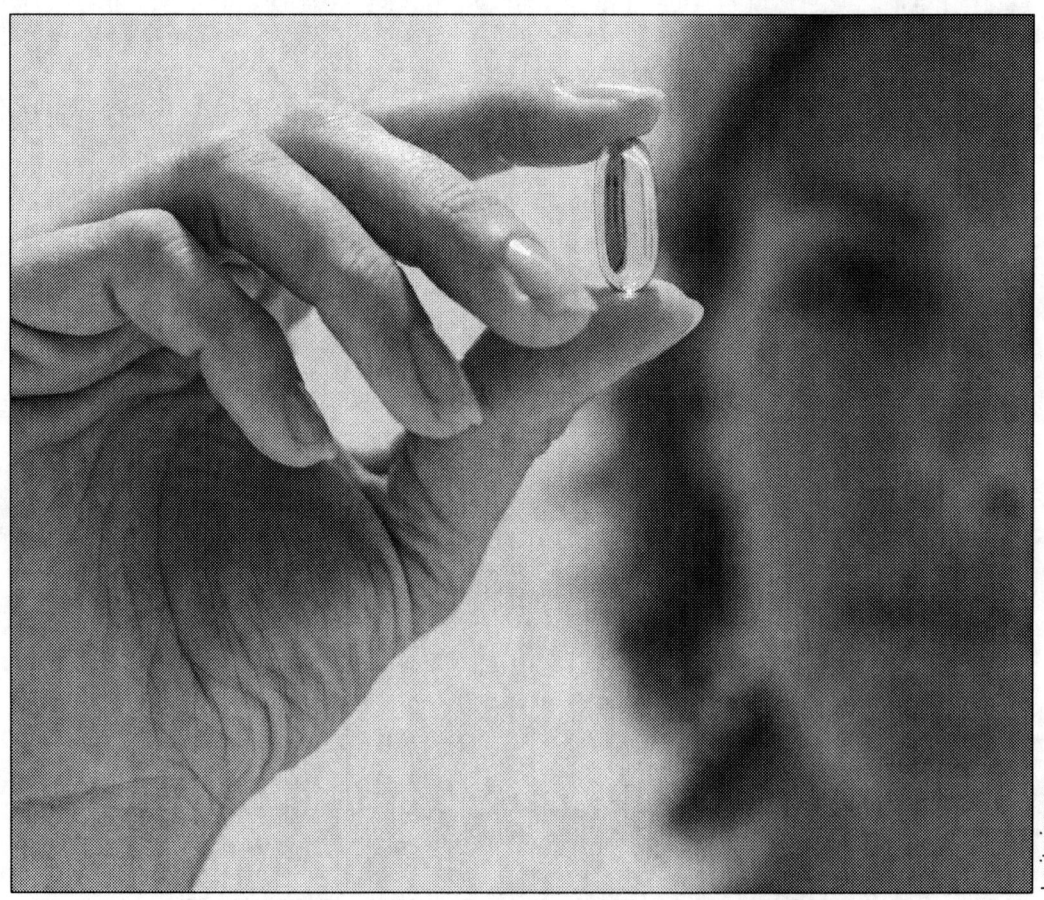

Eating SOD in pill form won't protect against free-radical damage or other oxidative stress in your body.

The "Stimulants and Sugar Water Are Health Food" Myth

Sales are high of sport products advertised as "giving energy." Technically, the potential energy in food is measured in units called calories. "High-energy snack" is a euphemism for "high-calorie food" or, in other words, "fattening food." Even though fat is stored energy, an obese individual will not automatically be energetic. An increasing number of sport products and "health food" contains stimulants such as caffeine, ginseng, or other substances.

Sugar helps delay fatigue if used during long endurance events where you can't stop to eat. For regular use, simple sugar is not health food, even though sold in "energy" and sport food. Simple sugars raise insulin levels, which drop soon after. Constant insulin production and circulation is not healthy. Complex carbohydrate mixed with a small amount of protein is often a better choice for nutrition for energy. You can do this with a piece of fruit and some raw nuts, like almonds or walnuts. For healthy energy, instead of relying on special energy foods, get good nutrition, keep your emotional health strong through practice, and get regular exercise.

The "Need It Now" Myth

Some sport-food advertising implies that, since vitamins and minerals are removed from your system by sporting activities, you need their specific foods that have those nutrients. General recreational exercise does not sufficiently deplete any nutrients to affect athletic ability or health. For that reason, after a one-hour hike or game of tennis, you don't need to replace specific vitamins or minerals immediately. Your next good meal will cover you. It is unnecessary to take extra vitamins or minerals ahead of time to offset any loss predicted during your exercise. You don't lose enough to affect performance or fatigue level. In general, regular, healthy eating and hydration assures you don't start your day in an already depleted state. Moreover, your daily requirements of most nutrients typically balance out over days. Minute-to-minute deficits don't matter as much.

Claim
- A common claim is that you are in danger of B12 deficiency if you don't eat red meat every day, or often, to replenish amounts you use each day.

Critical Reading
- Vitamin B12 is stored in your liver in enormous quantities, sufficient for years.

The "Reverse Reasoning" Myth

In this myth, if a deficit causes a weakness, then a surplus will bring strength. However, just as the right glasses prescription corrects vision, getting too strong a correction will not make you see better yet.

Vitamin E is a nutritional example. In experiments with rats years ago, researchers removed all Vitamin E from the rats' food. The rats became bald and sterile. Restoring Vitamin E restored the rats' hair and fertility. Marketing and advertising people used those results to launch campaigns to sell Vitamin E with claims of giving you hair and virility. Vitamin E does not do that for humans with adequate nutrition (but bald, sterile rats, take note).

Claims
- Vitamin A is often promoted as: "Needed for good night vision."
- High-calorie foods are often labeled as: "Giving you energy."
- Special powdered mixtures are advertised as: "Providing all the nutrients contained in healthy spinal discs," or containing "All the nutrients crucial to healthy hair."
- Free radicals are known to be involved in the various damage to the body caused by their oxidative nature. Vitamins C and E are known antioxidant agents against the oxidative free-radical activity. People often take extra Vitamins C and E on the presumption that it will reduce their risk of the various damaging effects of free radicals.

Critical Reading
- Vitamin A deficiency reduces ability to see in dim light. No amount of carrots or vitamin supplements will make adequately nourished eyes see better.
- Calorie deficiency makes you tired. Eating extra calories will not make you energetic. It will make you fat.
- Potions containing the nutrients or component substances of your back and hair don't fix your bad back or grow hair. They are regular food. Countless products line the shelves, stating they are for skin, nerves, strength, fingernails, or whatever—all just glamorized food. Your body needs specific nutrients to do its job, but eating more of them won't increase the processes.
- Vitamin E is lipid (fat) soluble and protects cell membranes, which have a major lipid component. Vitamin C is a water-soluble antioxidant, having protective effects in blood and the fluid inside and outside of cells. Vitamins E and C work together in their free radical inactivation work. The way Vitamin E inactivates radicals is to accept the extra electron that makes the molecules radical and reactive. When Vitamin E takes that extra electron, it becomes radical itself. Vitamin C then takes the extra electron from E to restore Vitamin E. Vitamin C is special in that it can accept this extra burden without injury to itself or surrounding molecules.

You need a minimum amount of these vitamins to do their jobs. It is true that many people, particularly those on a typical meat-eating Western diet, may not get enough Vitamins E and C, and many other disease-fighting antioxidants which are found in vegetables and fruits. Taking more of Vitamins E and C than you need has not been shown to increase their usual effects on radicals in the body. If you are vitamin deficient, they may help, but not if you are vitamin sufficient. Taking too much in isolated vitamin supplements may be injurious.

Free radicals are not all bad. Some perform critical functions in your body, such as muscle contraction and immune response. You may not want to push your resting levels down, even if it were possible to do so by eating antioxidants. If you got rid of the radicals stored in special cells in your body that fight infection, you would be at risk of catastrophic infections.

The "I Can Eat Anything I Want as Long as It Is Low-Fat (or Low-Carbohydrate)" Myth

Are you eating low-fat or low-carbohydrate diets and still not losing weight? Despite the claims about needing to eat fat for "zones" or fat burning, or that carbohydrates make you fat, it is the number of calories you eat of those "low-fat" foods compared to how much your lifestyle burns the calories. Low-fat cakes, cookies, and candies can easily be high-calorie and full of sugar.

A sack of sugar is non-fat, and a 1,000-calorie block of fat is sugar-free. Keep your common sense about you. Several hundred extra calories a day of "non-fat" or "low carbohydrate food" will store as fat.

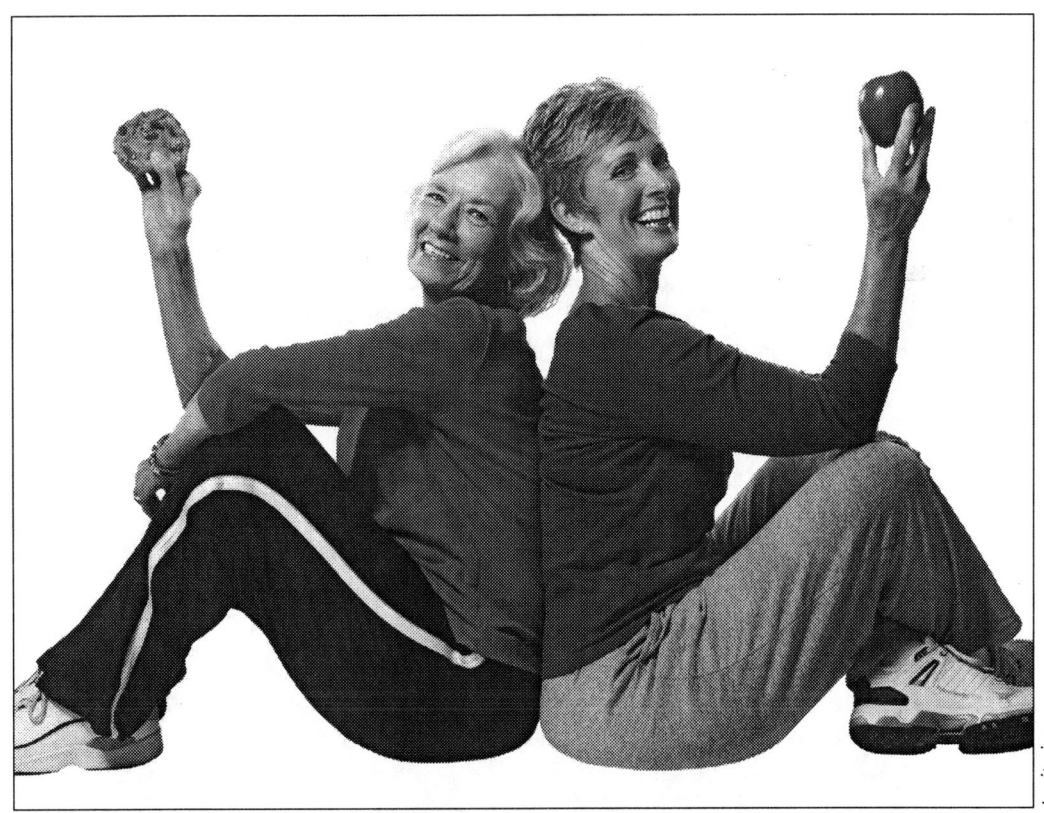

Despite the claims about needing to eat fat for "zones" or fat burning, or that carbohydrates make you fat, it is the number of calories you eat of those "low-fat" foods compared to how much your lifestyle burns the calories.

The "I Eat Right" Myth

An average person sits down to an evening meal of steak or burgers; potato mashed with butter, salt, and milk; coffee with cream and sugar; and a small side of buttered vegetables; then has ice cream and/or cake for dessert. A good dinner of protein for muscles, calcium for bones, and energy for exercise? No. The U.S. Department of Agriculture recently surveyed American dietary habits. The findings? Many Americans who think they eat healthy don't at all. The sample dinner is typical of three times too much fat, saturated fat, cholesterol, and salt; double the needed protein; too much simple sugar; insufficient fiber, vitamins, or complex carbohydrates; and not enough water. This kind of eating is increasingly associated with heart and vascular disease, vitamin deficiency, dehydration, calcium loss, high blood pressure, and some cancers.

The "Healthy Eating Is Awful" Myth

Why should low-fat, vegetable-based meals be called drastic, while cardiac bypass surgery, stroke, and colon cancer are considered normal? It is good news, not bad. Good meals need no secret energy foods and no special supplements. They can be good tasting and healthy in many ways and possibly cheaper than special health and sport performance foods.

Answers to Commonly Asked Questions

If the *Dietary Guidelines* and MyPlate are accurate, why is there an obesity problem in America?

The simplest answer to this question is that only a small percentage of the American population actually follows the guidelines. Many people consume excess energy and are physically inactive. In addition, many forces play a role in why Americans seem to have a steadily increasing waist circumference. We have access to food literally everywhere. We spend more time in our cars traveling and sitting idle in traffic than ever before. Schools identify physical education as a luxury that they cannot afford. Children are fascinated with inactive game consoles and electronics. City infrastructure limiting safe sidewalks and biking routes and perceived safety limitations make walking to school a challenge—and a story parents share with their children about a time long past. We seem to have advanced our culture to a place where physical activity and recreational enjoyment need specialized equipment and instruction, signed waivers, and significant participation fees, a situation that exists because communities no longer seem to value these activities—unless you can afford them. In other words, it's not just the Dietary Guidelines—that's only one piece of the equation.

How much of each nutrient does a person need?

Refer to the Dietary Reference Intakes (DRIs), which is a collaborative effort between the Food and Nutrition Board of the Institute of Medicine in the United States and Health Canada. DRIs are designed to meet the needs of approximately 97 to 98 percent of the healthy population. These recommendations may not be valid if a person has a disease or medical condition.

Why is it that many nutrition-related claims seem important today, but are gone in six months?

Often, the media will report the results of a single research study as fact. Sometimes, the person reporting does not pay attention to the study size or the statistical or clinical significance. A media headline is not the same as a government-issued dietary guideline or an abundance of scientific evidence.

How many calories does a person need?

Several ways of estimating energy expenditure are available. One method is a simple chart based on age, weight, and gender, while the other is a more complicated equation. Both methods provide estimates, but are good starting points. Actual energy needs may differ. If a person is consuming exactly the "required" amount of calories but is still gaining weight, then that estimated value is too high and needs to be adjusted.

If someone follows the MyPlate plan precisely, what would prevent him from losing weight?

First, the meal plan needs to include an energy deficit. If this is not specified, the plan will be created for weight maintenance. Second, the energy needs and meal plan that are presented on MyPlate are just an estimate. They provide a good starting point, but may need to be adjusted by the user. Third, consumers tend to underreport their serving sizes and total food intake. Underreporting is not usually purposeful, just a misunderstanding of portion sizes. People need to measure portion sizes at first and then can move away from this process once they become more proficient in judging portion sizes accurately. Estimating portion sizes gets easier when the same dishes are used (e.g., the same cereal bowl each morning). Finally, people do not always count items like hard candies, gum, small handfuls of snacks, or beverages that can add significant calories to the daily caloric intake.

What is the difference between foods that are enriched versus those that are fortified?

When grains are processed, many of the nutrients are lost. Enrichment is the process of adding back some of the nutrients lost with processing. Fortification is when a nutrient is added to a food that does not normally contain it. Examples are calcium-fortified orange juice or soy milk.

What is the difference between whole wheat and whole grain?

Whole grains are grains that are not refined—they are milled in their complete form with only the husk removed. Wheat flour is any flour made from wheat and may include unbleached flour or white flour. Whole-wheat bread, for example, may be brown in color due to lack of bleaching, but the fiber content may vary. To maximize fiber content in a product, look for the terms "whole grain" on the label.

Are carbohydrates bad?

First, carbohydrate (glucose) is necessary for the brain and other organs to function properly. If blood glucose falls too low, a coma can result. Carbohydrates also fuel the working muscle during exercise, with more fuel coming from carbohydrate as exercise intensity increases. Without adequate carbohydrate, exercise performance will suffer. It is important to understand the role of carbohydrate in fueling the skeletal muscle and organs.

Second, different qualities of carbohydrate are available. Many carbohydrate-rich foods (e.g., fruits, vegetables, and whole grains) contain fiber, vitamins, minerals, antioxidants, and phytochemicals. Eliminating these foods from the diet is not prudent for good health.

Carbohydrates will cause fat gain if more are eaten than are stored as glycogen or burned as fuel. Carbohydrates consumed in proper quantities will not promote weight gain. Think about elite distance runners—are they fat? No, even though they do consume large quantities of carbohydrate. Many sedentary individuals consume all macronutrients in excess, which leads to a positive energy balance and weight gain.

Insulin has been labeled by some as an undesirable anabolic hormone that promotes fat storage. It is true that it is anabolic, but it also plays a role in skeletal muscle protein synthesis. Insulin will promote fat storage if more carbohydrate is consumed than the body needs to replenish glycogen stores or use as fuel. If normal quantities of carbohydrate are eaten, the insulin response is not an important issue.

What is the relationship between oat fiber and lower cholesterol levels?

Commercials on television promote consumption of oat fiber to reduce serum cholesterol. Scientific data do support this claim—in fact, an FDA-approved health claim exists for the relationship (www.fda.gov). A key theory behind this observation involves the behavior of soluble fiber in the gastrointestinal tract. The soluble fiber acts as a sponge by absorbing some dietary fat consumed with a meal and by absorbing bile (a compound made in the liver and stored in the gallbladder that aids digestion). This filled sponge-like substance is not digested in the small intestine and is ultimately excreted by the body. As it is excreted, the fat and bile go with it. Under normal circumstances, bile in the small intestine is recycled and reused. Since some is lost with the excretion of fiber, the body needs to make more. A key compound needed for bile synthesis is cholesterol. The liver can get some cholesterol to make more bile from the bloodstream. This theory explains how blood cholesterol drops in response to regular consumption of oat fiber.

Why do some people supplement with B vitamins to prevent heart disease?

This new area of research has to do with the compound homocysteine. Homocysteine is an intermediate in normal protein metabolism and the Vitamins B6, B12, and folate play an important role in keeping this metabolic intermediate from building up. It is believed that high levels of homocysteine may cause arterial damage and, thus, contribute to the atherogenesis process. It is important to talk to a physician before supplementing with B vitamins to prevent heart disease.

Why do people take niacin to lower cholesterol?

Niacin is a B vitamin that when taken in pharmacological doses (> 50mg/day) may lower levels of low-density lipoprotein (LDL) and increase levels of high-density lipoprotein (HDL). Due to the media reporting of this research, many people are taking niacin for this purpose. The UL for niacin is 35mg per day, but many people are taking a gram or more. Unfortunately, though niacin may improve blood lipids, it may also cause liver problems and other undesirable side effects. It is important to talk to a physician before taking supplemental niacin to control blood lipids.

Are artificial sweeteners bad?

To describe any food or nutritional product as "bad" is limiting at best. Some foods are simply better than others. Artificial sweeteners are classified by the FDA as food additives (www.fda.gov). Similar to drugs, food additives must undergo years of testing before they are approved for use. Currently, all of the artificial sweeteners sold legally in the United States are approved for sale and use. The key word here is "artificial." These products are chemicals; however, their safety has been tested.

Where do ketones come from and are they good for weight loss?

Everybody makes ketones, but production increases with the consumption of low-carbohydrate diets. Carbohydrates are needed for the complete oxidation of a fatty acid molecule. If carbohydrate is limited, the normal pathway for fat breakdown is altered, and another pathway is available. The end product of this alternate pathway causes ketone production. Ketones are acids that alter the pH of the body when large amounts are accumulated. When people consume low carbohydrate diets, enough ketones are produced to cause side effects, including bad breath and appetite suppression, but generally people do not end up with a severe medical condition called ketoacidosis. In short, ketones come from the incomplete breakdown of fatty acids.

Why do people with diabetes sometimes develop ketoacidosis?

Ketoacidosis is common in people with uncontrolled type 1 diabetes. These individuals have plenty of carbohydrate (glucose) in the blood, but the glucose cannot enter the cells without insulin. As a result, the cells try to rely on fat for fuel, but fatty acids cannot be completely oxidized without carbohydrate and therefore ketones form. In this case, the levels can build up to the point where a person's body becomes so acidic that he can end up in a coma and die. This condition is serious and requires medical attention.

If a protein product has a biological value (BV) greater than 100 percent, is it superior to food?

Biological value compares the amount of nitrogen absorbed from the diet with that retained in body for maintenance and growth. Egg has a BV of 100 percent, meaning that 100 percent of the nitrogen that is absorbed is retained.

Many protein products are quite expensive, while foods like eggs and milk are not. Products that have a BV greater than 100 percent are not absolutely necessary; foods can still provide the body with all of the needed amino acids. If a person is worried that food has a lower BV than the newest supplement, taking an extra few bites of chicken or a few extra gulps of milk should compensate.

Is whey protein the best form of protein?

While a few studies have suggested that consumption of the branched-chain amino acids (leucine, isoleucine, and valine) aid in the post-exercise protein synthesis process, insufficient evidence exists to conclude that any particular type of protein is superior to others. Whey protein supplements get much attention due to their leucine content. Other foods are also good sources of leucine, including milk, tuna, and cottage cheese.

If too much protein is consumed, isn't the excess excreted in the urine?

Any amino acid that is not being used for protein synthesis, glucose synthesis, or ATP production is converted to a fatty acid and stored in the adipose tissue. In this process, it is true that the nitrogen from the amino acid will get converted to urea and excreted, but the carbon skeleton is not destroyed and is used to make a fatty acid. Consuming too many calories will result in body fat gain, even if the extra calories are in the form of protein.

Will consuming too much protein put too much stress on the kidneys?

It is true that the kidney must handle the nitrogen/urea from excess protein intake; however, it is not clear if this is a problem in people with healthy kidneys. People with renal disease cannot handle too much protein; but, this may not be the same case for healthy people. Until more research data are available, a confident answer to this question cannot be given. A lack of research data does not imply or guarantee safety.

Are protein needs met for a person who is practicing a vegan diet?

People who choose vegan diets consume no animal products, which are complete proteins. If a person who is a vegan consumes soy or has a wide variety of plant foods in the diet, it is possible to meet protein needs. Incomplete proteins (most plants) lack one or more essential amino acids, but can be combined to provide all of the essential ones (e.g., by combining rice and beans). The complementary foods do not have to be consumed in the same meal to get the benefits; a person can consume these foods throughout the day.

Do all people need to drink eight, 8-ounce glasses of water per day?

It is not clear where this "8 x 8" rule came from. While this recommendation may be appropriate for some people, fluid needs also depend on physical activity levels, environment, and sweat rate. Fluid recommendations also differ before, during, and after exercise.

Do fluid requirements need to be met with plain water or do all fluids count?

All fluids count toward the daily need, including water found in foods. Consuming all types of beverages, regardless of their sugar or caffeine content, will contribute to fluid needs.

Won't caffeinated beverages dehydrate?

While caffeine may be a diuretic, the current evidence suggests that it will not lead to dehydration as long as total fluid needs are met. The exception is when an individual is participating in physical activity and hydration needs are significant and rehydration capacity is challenged. When an individual is working out in a very hot environment, in a very cold environment, at a high altitude, or for more than 90 minutes, non-caffeinated beverages are preferred by many fitness trainers and medical professionals.

Is it better to consume a sport drink or water?

If a person is exercising at low or moderate intensity for 30 to 45 minutes, plain water is fine. Sport drinks are designed to replace the carbohydrate and electrolytes lost with higher exercise intensities that are continuous and last longer than 45 to 60 minutes or are intermittent in nature. A warm environment may also increase fluid and electrolyte needs and a sport drink may be appropriate in this situation.

Are commercial sport drinks needed, or can they be made at home?

Commercial sport drinks are formulated to replace the carbohydrate and electrolytes lost with exercise, and these formulas are based on abundant scientific research. The products are readily available and inexpensive, especially in the powdered form. If a person is completely against using a commercial sport drink, he could attempt to mimic the formula by mixing one cup of orange juice (or other juice with potassium) with one cup of water and adding 1/8 teaspoon of salt. This beverage will not contain the ideal mixture of carbohydrate sources (fructose, glucose, sucrose, glucose polymers), and the fructose alone in the juice may cause gastrointestinal stress.

Are fitness waters necessary? What are the benefits?

Fitness waters are lower in electrolytes and carbohydrate (3g per cup) than traditional sport drinks (14 to 15g per cup). Research supports increased fluid intake when the beverage tastes good. Some people need the fluid because they are exercising in a warm environment, but are not exercising intensely or long enough to warrant carbohydrate replacement. Fitness waters could be a desirable beverage in this situation. Caution should be used with excessive consumption if the water contains vitamins and minerals that have an upper limit established.

Are vitamin waters and energy bars necessary?

Many people purchase foods and beverages with added vitamins, minerals, and/or herbs not only for the calories, but because of the perceived benefit of consuming these foods. Many fortified products exist on the market today, from waters, to bars, to whole foods. If a person is consuming more than the upper limit for a nutrient, toxicity symptoms may result. Many people who consume fortified foods also may be taking vitamin and mineral supplements.

Will taking a vitamin and mineral supplement enhance performance?

If a person is not deficient in a vitamin or mineral, taking more will not enhance performance. While exercise may slightly increase the need for a few vitamins and minerals, the increased needs are small and can be met with the extra calories needed to support training.

Does exercise increase the production of free radicals?

Free radicals are molecules that are thought to cause cellular damage. Antioxidant nutrients neutralize these free radicals in the body and are, therefore, recommended in the diet. Exercise will increase free radical production, but it also induces the synthesis of the body's antioxidant enzymes. It is believed that exercise does not contribute to the free-radical-induced damage thought to play a role in aging or chronic disease.

Can anybody change his body shape with appropriate nutrition and exercise?

While all nutrition and fitness professionals agree that proper nutrition and exercise are important for maintaining a healthy body composition, not everybody can significantly alter his body shape. Genetics plays a large role in body types. Some individuals who are tall and lean may never have the physique of a competitive bodybuilder. Similarly, individuals who are naturally larger may never be able to "diet" or train enough to become an elite marathon runner.

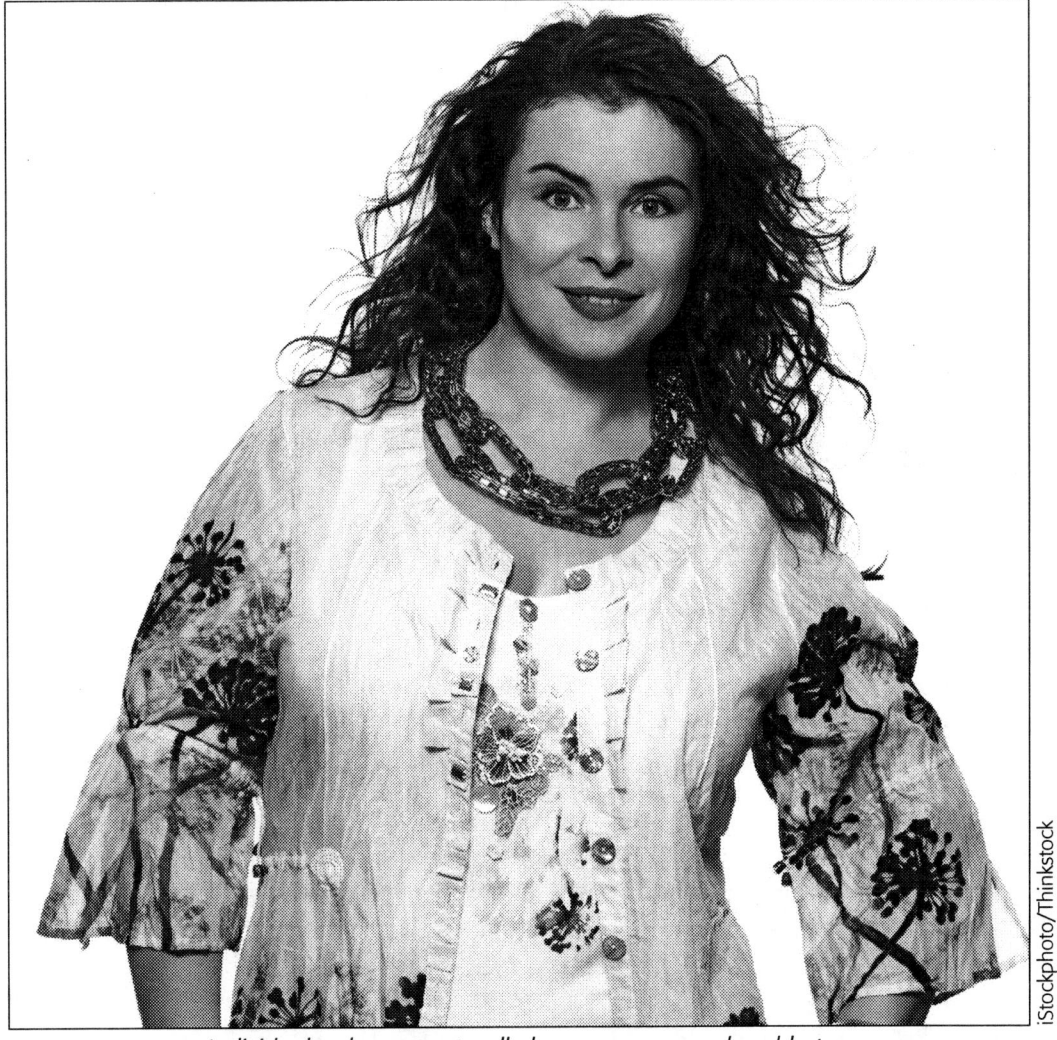

Individuals who are naturally larger may never be able to "diet" or train enough to become an elite marathon runner.

How is weight gained?

Most people asking this question are looking to increase muscle mass, not gain body fat. In order to gain muscle a person must have a positive energy balance and perform resistance training. Generally, an additional 400 to 500 kcals/day are needed, including adequate protein for strength training (1.5 to 2.0g/kg).

Will eating several smaller meals in a day stimulate metabolism?

Some scientific data supports the idea that multiple smaller meals spread throughout the day are better than two or three larger meals because the smaller meals "keep the furnace burning" or, more technically, increase the thermic effect of food. The magnitude of the additional calories burned is not very high (i.e., maybe 25 calories per day). Though the value may be small, it can add up over a period of time.

Smaller meals may contribute to successful weight loss and maintenance in another way. If a long period of time passes between meals, blood glucose levels may drop, which triggers fatigue and hunger. This physiologically driven hunger may result in overeating at the next meal. By keeping blood glucose level throughout the day, the highs and lows of blood sugar can be prevented and hunger better controlled.

Does metabolism slow down with age?

Research data suggest that as people age, a significant loss of skeletal muscle mass takes place due to physical inactivity. Unfortunately, resting metabolic rate may also decline in proportion to the muscle mass loss. The good news is that several research studies have reported that previously sedentary older adults respond well to resistance training and are capable of increasing both strength and muscle mass.

Will eating at certain times of the day promote weight gain?

Many diet plans will make recommendations that include no consumption of carbohydrates past 3:00 p.m. or no food at all past 7:00 p.m. This issue can be examined in two ways. From a physiological and digestive standpoint, the body does not know what time it is. Food can be digested with the same efficiency in the morning as in the evening. One of the claims in support of this idea is that eating before bed leads the food to be stored as fat. This is true, but the whole picture needs to be examined. The body is chronically storing fat in the adipose tissue and breaking it down when needed. In other words, just because a meal is stored as fat does not mean that it will remain in the adipose tissue forever. If a large evening meal is consumed and then used for fuel during a morning workout, it will not contribute to significant weight gain in the long term. If that large evening meal is not used for fuel, it may contribute to permanent body fat mass. The main concern here is long-term energy balance over several days, not just in a 12-hour period.

Another factor that is valid about meal timing has to do with behavior. If a person who is trying to lose weight skips meals, he may often end up excessively hungry in the evening, which could trigger the consumption of an enormous dinner. In this case, it is better to balance out food intake throughout the day to prevent overeating at one meal.

Finally, many occupations involve people working evening shifts. If a person gets off work at 11:00 p.m. or 3:00 a.m., is he supposed to not eat? As long as energy balance is maintained over the long term, the actual time of day does not matter.

Do the calories from beverages need to be counted?

Yes! Many popular smoothie shops and coffee houses offer drinks that can have several hundred calories. In addition, a can of soda has an average of 150 calories. Many people do not think about this since it is just a beverage and not a chewable food.

How can the status of bone health be determined?

When people go for a physical exam, often physicians will order blood work. While this practice is very useful in determining disease risk or diagnosing many diseases, it is not helpful for measuring bone health. While approximately 99 percent of the body's calcium is in bone, the remainder is in the blood and is essential for muscle contraction. Serum calcium is maintained within a very narrow window. If it drops just a bit, muscle contraction (e.g., heart beat) can be disrupted. When serum calcium drops, the calcium from bone can be used to restore the normal level. If a person's endocrine system is working properly, serum calcium will always be normal. The best way to evaluate the density of bones is through dual-energy x-ray absorptiometry (DXA or DEXA). This procedure usually requires a physician's order.

Are people genetically destined to be overweight or obese?

Genetics plays a large role in overweight and obesity. American society implies that ultrathin is the norm. Some people, no matter how much they control their food intake and exercise, will never be thin, and this is perfectly acceptable. However, people should not use the excuse of a family history of obesity to give up and not even bother to live a healthy lifestyle. For example, if a female is 5'4" tall, weighs 220 pounds, and has obese parents, it is hard to determine whether her obesity is due to lifestyle or genetics, but at the same time this is not that important. This person may never weigh the "ideal" 120 pounds due to genetic factors. However, with lifestyle modification, she may be able to weigh 150 or 160 pounds. It is important to determine a healthy body weight and to focus on fitness.

Why do some people on high animal-fat diets lower their cholesterol levels?

If people follow a low-carbohydrate, high-fat diet properly, they will lose some weight because such diets generally are low in calories. When a person loses weight, serum cholesterol levels will generally drop, no matter how the weight was lost. Limited research data are available examining the long-term effects of low-carbohydrate, high animal-fat diets on blood lipids or incidence of heart disease.

How much exercise is necessary for weight loss and weight maintenance?

The amount of exercise necessary for weight loss and weight maintenance is more than that recommended for good health. Data from the National Weight Control Registry, a large research trial examining successful weight loss and maintenance, indicate that 90 percent of the successful members exercise about one hour per day. The women had an average weekly energy expenditure of approximately 2,500 calories, while the men expended approximately 3,900 calories. Other data suggest that 60 to 90 minutes per day of accumulated physical activity is necessary for weight maintenance, with an energy expenditure goal of at least 2,000 calories per week. It is important to find activities that you will perform on a regular basis.

If an individual reduces the risk factors for disease, is he then safe?

Many health campaigns promote knowing personal numbers. This advice may apply to blood lipids, blood pressure, or blood glucose. It is important to understand the relationship between risk factors and disease development. For example, dyslipidemia is a risk factor for developing cardiovascular disease and hypertension is a risk factor for having a stroke. However, people with normal blood lipids or blood pressures can develop these conditions. Having positive risk factors significantly increases the likelihood of developing disease, but not having those risk factors does not preclude a person from ever getting a particular disease.

How much weight loss is needed to see health benefits?

Some overweight and obese people believe that they must achieve some unrealistic, "ideal" body weight in order to receive any health benefits. Fortunately, many people with chronic disease symptoms—such as elevated blood lipids, blood glucose, or blood pressure—can see improvements with modest weight loss of approximately 10 percent of body weight. Use this information to make those small steps toward improving health.

Does a person burn more fat when exercising at low intensity?

During low-intensity exercise, a greater percentage of the total calories come from fat. However, more total fat calories can be burned by higher-intensity exercise. When two,

20-minute exercise bouts are compared, one at lower intensity and one at higher intensity, the lower intensity bout expends 100 calories—80 percent from fat (i.e., 80 fat calories). At the higher intensity, 200 calories are burned, and only 50 percent are from fat, or 100 fat calories. If time is not a factor, a person could exercise for a longer duration at the lower intensity and burn the same number of total fat calories. On the other hand, lower-intensity exercise does not provide the same degree of cardiovascular benefits as moderate- or high-intensity exercise.

What is the difference between glycemic index and glycemic load?

Glycemic index (GI) is defined as the incremental area under the plasma glucose curve in response to 50 grams of available carbohydrate, in the fasted state, as compared to a reference food (glucose or white bread). In simple terms, it is a rating scale of a food's potential to raise blood glucose levels. A food with a "high" GI may cause large fluctuations in blood glucose. Initially, a large rise in blood glucose may occur, followed by a large increase in insulin secretion, which then may result in a dramatic fall in blood glucose concentrations.

Glycemic load (GL) is the amount of total carbohydrate in a food multiplied by the GI of the carbohydrate in that food. A normal portion of food may have a high GI, but a low GL.

Is it better to use glycemic index or glycemic load?

Either method should be used as a tool, not a rule. This information is useful if the body needs glucose quickly. In this case, choosing a high-GI food or product is appropriate. However, the GI should not always be a rule, especially when people believe they need to avoid certain foods. For example, carrots have a relatively high GI (~68) for a vegetable, but the GL is approximately 3. Learning the limitations of GI and GL and knowing your own body response is important.

Are there other factors that affect the glycemic index of a food?

Many factors may affect the GI of a food. Examples include the following: changes in particle size (e.g., mashing a potato); cooking; variety (e.g., a potato grown in Canada versus Idaho); maturation and ripening; addition of protein (e.g., adding chicken and cheese to a baked potato); and variability within foods (e.g., ice cream may have a GI of 35 to 65).

What are functional foods?

Functional foods are those that provide health benefits because of the compounds they contain beyond the traditional nutrients. For example, many fruits and vegetables contain phytochemicals, which are nonnutritive compounds with apparent health benefits.

What are probiotics and prebiotics?

Probiotics are examples of functional foods that contain live microorganisms that occur naturally or are added to the food. Their purpose is to promote a positive bacterial environment in the intestines. Prebiotics are non-digestible fibers that promote the growth of the beneficial gut bacteria. Prebiotics may occur naturally or may be added to a food.

What is exercise-induced hyponatremia, and how can it be avoided?

Exercise-induced hyponatremia is a condition where plasma sodium falls to a level than can be dangerous. The most common cause of this condition is when a person loses significant amounts of sodium through sweat loss and replaces the lost fluid with plain water. This condition can be avoided by consuming appropriate amounts of fluid and sodium to match the amount lost in sweat. Many sport drinks and products are readily available and can be used to prevent this condition.

Is drinking soda bad for the bones?

The mineral phosphorus is an important component of the hydroxyapatite found in bones (provides harness to bone tissue). Phosphorus is found in many common foods, including milk, meats, and eggs. Phosphoric acid is found in many soft drinks. A few studies have suggested an association between soft drink consumption and reduced bone mass. The proposed theories for this association were the following:
- Consuming soft drinks in place of milk leads to a decreased calcium intake.
- The acid and phosphorus in the soft drinks results in increased calcium loss.
- Caffeine in soft drinks results in increased calcium loss.

More recent studies suggest that it is likely the inadequate calcium consumption rather than intake of phosphorus or caffeine that leads to reduced bone mass.

CHAPTER 2
HEALTHY
WEIGHT-MANAGEMENT HABITS

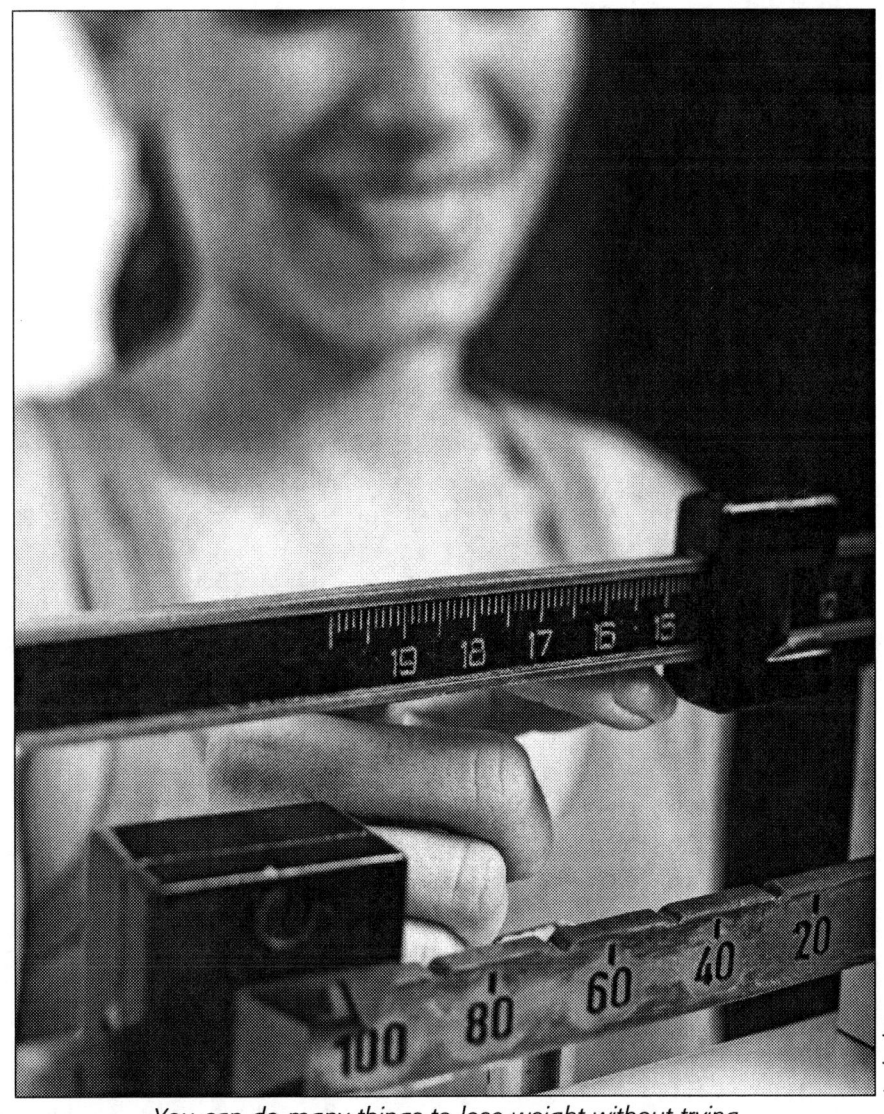

You can do many things to lose weight without trying unhealthy fad diets or eating foods you hate.

Let's make sure everyone understands that fat is not bad. Yes, we said it, fat is not bad. In fact, everyone requires a certain amount of body fat for warmth, cushioning, buoyancy in water, long-term energy requirements, and overall good health. However, it's also no secret that the average American has too much fat as part of their total body composition. A common health message heard from your doctor, from the magazine article that you are reading, from a conversation with coworkers, or from your spouse is "you need to lose weight to improve your health." Maintaining your body fat percentage at a healthy level has been associated with reducing the incidence of cardiovascular disease, metabolic disorders, orthopedic limitations, and even the psychological stress we all feel at one time or another. The purpose of this chapter is not to tell you to reduce your level of fat to a predetermined percentage of your total body weight. The purpose of this chapter is to explain the habits that are associated with achieving a healthy balance of fat percentage to total body weight and the weight management techniques people have found to be successful and reproducible.

You can do many things to lose weight without trying unhealthy fad diets or eating foods you hate. It is not enough to say, "I'll lose 10 pounds by next month." Get started by taking a clear look at the way you eat now and how much activity you get on a daily basis.

It's Not Metabolism

Many false claims are made about metabolism. Metabolism is seldom the culprit with regard to weight gain. Are you eating more than you used to in past years, exercising less, doing less, sitting around more, and eating junk food, snack food, fast food, and soda? Weight gain associated with these behaviors is *not* a slowing of your metabolism due to aging.

The fact that you burn fewer calories when you decrease activity can be twisted by clever product advertising as "slower metabolism." Don't fall for it. Find fun, healthy things you like to do, and start doing them again to get the increase in metabolic calorie burning that comes with activity.

Don't fall for pills and supplements advertised to increase metabolism and, therefore, promote weight loss. Some products contain stimulating compounds that increase heart rate or other functions, which is not helpful or healthy for your body. Many people feel stimulated and happy on these products, and don't notice the nervousness, anxiety, inability to focus, moodiness, difficulty falling asleep at night, and depression which also often occurs. A more serious cycle starts when people take other drugs to try to stop these symptoms—and then more drugs when the first drugs upset their stomach. Exercise will improve your mood and increase your metabolism for weight loss more safely without the negative effects of stimulants and medicines.

Eating food raises metabolism? The increase comes because your body has to do something extra: digestion. You still gain calories from the food you consume and can gain weight if you eat more calories than you burn. Watch out for advertising that exploits the laws of "thermogenics" (heat-producing or calorie-burning) effect of food. The effect is small compared to the calories you have eaten.

Some devices and pills claim to increase metabolism even after exercise ends. They can claim so because all exercise has that effect—with or without the device or pill. Exercise raises metabolic levels. It takes time after stopping exercise to return to resting level.

Change Unhealthful Eating Habits

A British study conducted in 2006 found that exercise alone won't prevent childhood obesity. The children in one of the groups got exercise, but didn't lose weight because they were eating more calories than they burned. They still received several health benefits of exercise plus important motor skills. However, the message is that if you eat more calories than you need, it can become extra weight, of course. Changing unhealthy eating is needed, too.

More calories than you use each day results in more weight. An easy way to improve weight and health at the same time is to stop eating junk. It is called junk for a reason. Don't give children soda or diet soda any more than you would give them cigarettes. People may say, "You have to let them have a little fun," or, "If I don't let them have a little, they will want it more." Would you say the same about heroin? Antifreeze tastes sweet, too, but children are taught not to drink it because it is harmful. Talk to them. Teach them a better way. Set an example of exercising strength by putting away the cookies and shakes. Don't eat the 1,000-calorie bag of chips. Do fun exercise with them like catch, skipping rope, tumbling, and fun games you make yourself. Please do not tell your friends that this book recommends that you never eat a cookie or drink a shake. All that is being recommended is common sense and moderation. If you're not sure how much that is, then it's probably less than you think it is.

Remember that children can't wait to run away from the table to play, but are directed into the habit of sitting still and eating everything on their plate. Don't make them hold still when they can run. These common practices teach them to be sedentary overeaters who have too much pent-up energy to concentrate in school or sleep at night. Let them jump and play after dinner instead of sitting in front of a television. Tell them how happy you are to be together, but then go play. If they have homework to complete, the scientific literature is clear: kids perform better in their schoolwork after they have participated in large muscle physical activities.

Some people say they don't have money to eat healthful food, yet spend the same money and more on junk food, supplements, "calming" drugs, and "energy" drinks. Put the money in a jar and exercise instead, and you can lose weight and feel calm plus feed the poor. Sport drinks with refined sugar and stimulant compounds are not healthy for everyday life or for exercise. Eat a banana instead. It is not more time-consuming or difficult to steam or sauté in balsamic vinegar and spices instead of fry. It can be fun, not worrisome, to try something that will easily help your health. You don't need to buy a steamer; use any pot. Put any cut washed vegetables that you like in the pot with a small amount of water, balsamic or other cooking vinegar, and seasonings. Put the lid on, and the heat will steam them in the seasoned broth. It takes not much more time than it takes to open a can of processed soup with too much salt, fillers, unhealthy fats, sweeteners, and little fiber or vitamins left after processing. The rest of this chapter offers healthy things to do instead of old counterproductive habits.

Reduce Fat and Refined Sugar

Reduce extra fat in your diet to reduce unhealthful calories so you can lose weight. Some high-fat diets result in weight loss because of few total calories; however, it is not a healthful way to lose weight. Eating less saturated fat and trans-fat reduces risk of heart disease, diabetes, and some cancers.

According to some studies, cutting back extra fat is a better way to lose weight than cutting only calories. Some of the reasoning for this idea is that your body uses fewer calories to digest fat than it does to digest carbohydrate. The human body is designed to store fat, and more easily stores it when provided directly. It does not mean to eat sugary junk food and refined white flour, which is little more than junk food. Refined flour and sugar products like toast and crackers and cookies can raise your blood fat as much as eating fatty food.

Many foods may be high fat, but because they also have so much sugar, the overall percentage of fat on the label seems low. Don't be fooled. Take a good, hard look at what you eat and where all the extra calories are coming from.

> **A low fat percentage on the food label doesn't always mean the item is low in fat. It may be full of fat, but have so many calories from sugar that the proportion is low by comparison.**

Make Your Own

Many common prepared "convenience" foods are just not healthy. They also cost more than making your own healthy foods. Making your own food doesn't have to take time. It often can be quicker than stopping for convenience foods.
- For a quick breakfast, instead of sugared cereal with milk and a toaster pastry, have fruit and some raw nuts (like walnuts and almonds). People with tree nut and peanut allergy can often eat seeds like sunflower.
- If you want cereal in a bowl, put oats in a bowl, add a few sunflower seeds, walnuts, almonds, or pumpkin seeds, and cinnamon. Pour in hot water and stir. You can add dozens of other healthy things, from homemade almond milk, to apples and

bananas, to other quick grains like millet or brown rice. For simple, no-grain breakfast, put fruit pieces in a bowl with raw nuts and some cinnamon.

- For quick meals in a glass, throw water in a blender, and add any combination of hundreds of healthy foods. Add raw nuts, apple slices (with the skin), peeled orange slices, apricots, flax seeds (the blender will mill them), sesame seeds, pumpkin seeds, grapes, carrots, or blueberries. Other flavor possibilities are unsweetened vanilla bean or unsweetened powdered baking cocoa. Make as thick or thin as you like. Drink and go. Pack some in clean, safe containers to go for a lunch drink instead of soda.
- Replace commercial soda with your own. Squeeze a lemon or lime into a glass of carbonated or non-carbonated water. Throw fruit in a blender with a little water. Once blended, add seltzer to the consistency you want.
- Instead of processed peanut butter and refined sugar jelly, put fresh, raw peanuts (or other favorites, like walnuts) in a bowl and crush them for arm exercise with any kitchen pounding tool, or use a chopper, grinder, blender, coffee grinder, or other processor. Crush to powder, depending how chunky you want it. Mash in apple cubes to make moist, creamy sweet peanut butter. Spice with cinnamon if you want. In less than a minute of preparation time, you have a sweet nut butter that you can spread on fruit slices, carrots, and other good foods. Make it portable by stuffing inside raw sweet green and red peppers, in sandwich and wraps (non-grain eaters can make tasty wraps from leafy greens). Use for toppings. Vary the combinations; try almonds mashed with pears, sunflower seeds or walnuts and banana, or sesame seeds and figs. Make with a friend for healthy, social fun.
- Make your own sprouts. Put dry mung beans on a shallow plate and cover with water, or use any beans like small red beans, or seeds like clover. Each day or so, rinse the beans and replace the water. They will sprout in a few days. Rinse well, and throw in a pan when you sauté vegetables. Season to taste. Eat them when only a few days sprouted for nuttier taste, or wait for longer growth for more vegetable taste.
- Instead of refined-sugar sport drinks, put a peeled whole cucumber into a food processor, mixer, or low-speed blender with a whole kiwi fruit. It will make a sweet, cool, slushy, green drink.
- Make your own sweet drinks by putting a red sweet pepper in any kind of food grinder, masher, or blender. Cut about an inch of fresh ginger root and add through the grinder. In about 30 seconds preparation time, you will have a sweet, cool, red, slushy drink with an exotic tang of ginger. It is healthy and good tasting.

Substitute

Substitute a lower-calorie for a higher-calorie food, and healthy food for junk. When you are about to eat foods full of refined sugar and fat, eat something better instead—an apple, a pear and some walnuts, a roasted, seasoned sweet potato without any junk sauce. Complex carbohydrates used to be called starches and were avoided. Eating sensible amounts of complex carbohydrates, rather than too much fat and simple sugar, is a key to healthier eating. Main good sources are fruit and vegetables for daily meals. Use moderate amounts of legumes like lentils and whole grains to fuel exercise. Be creative, and find things you like.

For Snacks

- For a cold treat without unhealthy junk food, mash a frozen banana with crushed raw walnuts or flax seeds. Use a food grinder, or get free exercise by mashing them yourself in a bowl. It will taste like creamy ice cream.
- Have raisins and grapes instead of candy. Not too much of these, though, since they are sugary. Brush your teeth after eating raisins. The sugar sticks to your teeth.
- Have bananas with cinnamon instead of banana cake.
- Have an apple and walnuts instead of cinnamon buns or donuts.
- Many brands of fruit-flavored yogurts contain fruit jam, adding the equivalent of eight or nine teaspoons of sugar per cup. If you eat dairy, use or make plain yogurt, and add your own fresh fruit.
- Try chili powder and other seasonings instead of butter on air-popped popcorn. Use either multi-spice chili powder seasoning or the ground powder of chile peppers (e.g., chipotle or ancho). Make sure any seasoning you use does not have added sugar, MSG, or other additives.
- Have dry-roasted and raw nuts like almonds and walnuts instead of roasted, honey-roasted, or salted nuts. Remember not to sit watching television while eating a can of honey-roasted nuts, which can total over 1,000 calories. Don't eat many cups of nuts a day; they are not low calorie, just a healthier food than processed snack food.
- Drink juice with the pulp. Processed grape juice, for example, is a common sweetener put in factory foods to masquerade as "healthy." It is little more than sugar water. Put fruit in a blender or other mixer or grinder with clean water rather than purchase commercial juice.
- Instead of chips, pretzels, and dip at your next party, serve cut sweet peppers; grapes, strawberries, olives, and other easy finger fruit; raw nuts (not honeyed); and cubed, baked sweet potato and roasted or pan-sautéed zucchini. Use chopped hot-pepper salsa and unsweetened applesauce (easy recipe in this chapter) for dip.
- For holiday parties and Halloween giveaways, try bags of oranges and apples, notepads to write thoughts, walnuts in the shell to crack for hand strength, individual-size cans of fun clay to sculpt with, inexpensive eye-hand coordination toys, and other healthful fun treats.
- To make sweet herbal teas, try cinnamon, cloves, grated orange peel, or ginger in hot water.

For Cooking

- Bake, sauté, and steam instead of fry. You don't need to buy a steamer. Put your favorite vegetables in the bottom of any saucepan with an inch or so of water, depending on the pot size. Sprinkle balsamic vinegar, seasonings, and a small amount of olive oil over the top, and put the lid on to steam until tender.
- Put olive oil or grape seed oil in a misting bottle to make your own non-stick spray, or wipe half a teaspoon of oil around the pan using a towel, brush, or hand.
- Use seasonings instead of butter. Seasonings have antioxidant and other healthful properties. Try packaged, ground seasonings such as curry, ginger, pepper, oregano, and others. Then, try grating fresh ginger root and turmeric using any ordinary hand-held grater. Fresh ginger and turmeric root is available in produce sections many grocery stores. Turmeric is a principle ingredient in curry, and researched for anti-cancer properties, but don't overdo turmeric; just season with it. Try fresh green mint, oregano, basil, and cilantro leaves in vegetables and soup.
- Steam and sauté using soup stock instead of oil; roast and braise in balsamic vinegar and seasonings instead of fat.
- Grind plain sea salt instead of using packaged salt, which often contains chemicals against caking, and other agents. Practice adding and using less salt to meals.
- Use aromatic foods to flavor sauces instead of butter, cream, or cheese. Aromatic foods include tomatoes, onions, garlic, mushrooms, leeks, fresh parsley, thyme, oregano, and basil. Many aromatics have been found to have high antioxidant and other health benefits.
- Refrigerate soups and stocks to separate and congeal the fat, skim it off, and use the skimmed product instead.
- Use whole grains, not white-flour pastas. Use brown and wild rice, not white rice. Don't overdo grains. They are nutrient-dense and best for days of exercise and exertion. Eat fewer grains when doing less exercise.

For Meals

- Roasting vegetables caramelizes the natural sugar. Roast sweet peppers with onions, mushrooms, and green vegetables. No need to peel the skins. The skins have healthful nutrients. Brush with vinegar or tomato sauce to marinade. Season with any number of healthy seasonings.
- Instead of pouring oil on salad, try balsamic vinegar, pureed cucumbers, seasonings, and hot sauce. Seasoned Japanese rice-wine vinegar tastes sweet and rich enough to seem like oil. Make vinaigrette with healthy grape seed oil.
- Instead of cream on a potato, try lemon-pepper seasoning (without MSG or additives), real brewed soy sauce, hot pepper, horseradish, or wasabi. Prepare it so you can eat the skin, too.

- When you cook vegetables, don't use sugar, butter, cream, or sauce. Throw in onion, scallions, chives, shallots, nuts (like sunflower seeds and almonds), and hot peppers, and season with ginger, tamari, garlic, or curry.
- Make brown rice with lentils, peanuts, barley, green beans, peas, onions (or leeks), and hot sauce. Cook rice in fresh peaches with ginger. Cook in unsweetened pineapple and curry. Try tamari sauce. It is different every time.
- Put soft, cooked sweet potato in many foods you want to make sweet—your morning hot cereal, the morning blender drink, afternoon sandwiches, pies, baked goods, rice, or lentils. Make it sweeter with apples or spicy with onions. Don't overdo. Sweet potato still has calories. Don't add sugar glaze or butter. Good for days of high activity.
- You may be surprised how good onions can taste cooked with a sweet vegetable.
- You can do a lot with mangoes. They can sweeten vegetables, both cooked and raw. Mix chili peppers and mashed mango pulp into a sweet and tangy sauce. It is easy and fast.
- Substitute lentil and vegetable dinners for meat. With all the fruit, vegetables, legumes, beans, and grains available, you can eat a different, healthful, good tasting meal every day.

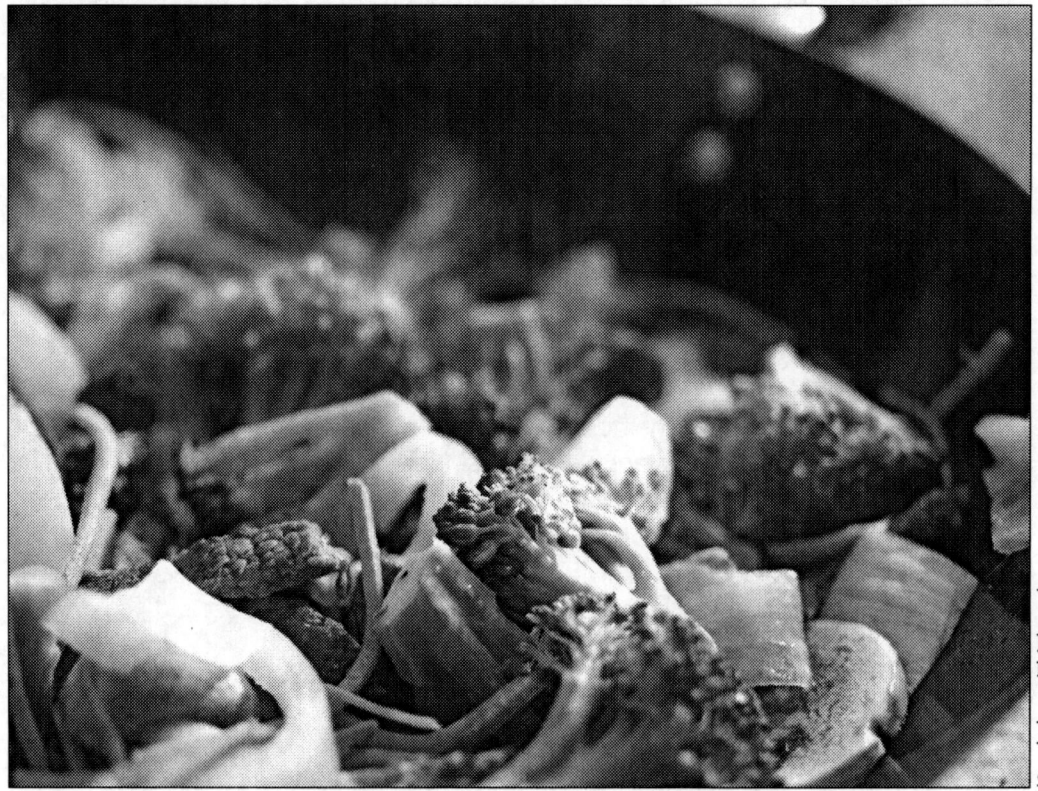

When you cook vegetables, don't use sugar, butter, cream, or sauce.

For Baking

Common baking recipes use large amounts of fat and sugar. Your baking can be sweet and moist without the cholesterol-raising kinds of fat, sugar, or eggs.

- Mash apples, bananas, or soaked prunes and substitute them for most or all oil and sugar. Substitute approximately 1:1 by volume, or experiment on your own.
- Use walnuts milled in your blender or pounded to powder in a bowl, instead of oil and eggs.
- Add a sweet potato instead of oil or sugar for creamy, moist, good taste.
- For icing, spread fresh mashed apples (homemade applesauce) easily made in a bowl using a pounder, or putting fresh apple slices in a blender. Use edible flowers or even (non-edible) real or plastic flowers as decoration instead of icing.
- Instead of taking a cake-decorating class, take a decorative vegetable–carving class, or get a book and try your own.

For Desserts

- For sweet desserts, try fruit and frozen, whole-juice popsicles instead of pie and ice cream. Make your own whole juice in a blender instead of drinking sugar water in commercial juices. For a simple dessert, chew fresh green mint leaves.
- Quickly make your own applesauce without added sugar or syrup. Cut apples into manageable cubes and mash them in a bowl to get exercise, or put whole apples into a grinder. Add cinnamon or nutmeg. Use over oatmeal instead of sugar, and over fruit for dessert and snacks.
- Make baked apple with cinnamon instead of sugar or honey. It will be sweet.
- Instead of ice cream, it is quick and easy to make your own frozen dessert. Add a scoop of unsweetened baking cocoa to a frozen mashed banana and crushed walnuts for a healthy sweet wonderful treat that tastes better than you would expect. For exotic flavor and more health benefit, add fresh grated ginger root. Real unsweetened cocoa (not processed, sweetened, chocolate candy) is a healthful food. It contains theobromine, an antioxidant, weak diuretic, stimulant, and mood booster. Compounds in cocoa open breathing airways and relieve coughing. Dark chocolate has more theobromine than lighter chocolate, with flavonoids and phenolics, plant substances that are good for the heart. People who get a kind of vascular headache called migraine do better not to eat chocolate.
- Substitute talking with your friends, or stretching, or appreciating the dinner centerpiece instead of eating dessert.
- Dessert does not have to be simple sugar and fat. Something can be good for you and still be a treat.

Don't Go Hungry

It is not true that dieting makes you fat because you get hungry and eat more. If you eat more, that is your decision. The idea is to be happy eating healthful things, not to be hungry and unhappy. Eating junk food and eating too frequently can keep insulin levels too high in the body, which is not healthy and can make you feel you want to eat. Relax and enjoy changing to healthier habits. Stand up straight over the counter with shoulders back to cut sweet peppers for snacks, instead of hunching over a bag of chips.

Don't just eat "low-fat" cakes, cookies, and sweets. They are full of simple sugar, which will make you hungry within a few hours—usually sooner. Get protein from nuts, seeds, grains, vegetables, and legumes like lentils.

Eat Less Simple Sugar

Simple or refined sugar is just about everywhere in prepared foods. The label may say "no sugar," "natural," or "organic," but don't be fooled. They can be full of refined empty-calorie sweeteners, like dextrose, high-fructose corn syrup, maltose, grape juice, rice syrup, galactose, and in refined flour products in crackers, biscuits, bread, and other processed foods that don't list added sugar.

Eat complex carbohydrates like fruit, red peppers, and brown rice for snacks instead of candy. Don't eat donuts and Danish or packaged cereal for breakfast. When you stop eating sugar, a magic thing happens: you crave less. Keep a list if you have to, to see what you eat every day. Find out where all the extra sugar you eat is coming from. You will save money and your health by not buying prepared snack foods. They are not good for you.

Don't buy candy or cakes or keep them in the house. They are refined sugar and hydrogenated fat. Don't give them to children. It is not parental love. It is the same as giving them cigarettes or addictive drugs. Change that. Parental love is giving them beautifully functioning, self-control brain centers.

Be Prepared

Food away from home at fast-food places, restaurants, the workplace, public events, and snack machines are high-fat, high-sugar, high-calorie, and low in nutrition. Go prepared. Pack fruit, sliced sweet peppers, and nuts to snack on, so you don't wind up with fries, shakes, and candy. Pack a brown rice and lentil lunch (cooked without oil or cream sauces) mixed with vegetables and seasonings, rather than oil.

Avoid most commercial sport nutrition bars and drinks. They are no more than candy with a sporty name. Sport bars and drinks are not magic energy potions; they are regular food, and often junk food, in a wrapper.

Improve Your Mindset

A better body and spirit come more from healthful movement in daily life than from an eating disorder. Stop eating junk soda and candy because you want to be healthier, and practice having control, instead of acting on every impulse.

It is not being a good parent to give young children candy any more than it is being a good parent to give them cigarettes. To be a good parent, give them self control and good self-image though healthy lifetime habits.

Involve the People You Cook For

If you cook for people who don't eat healthful meals or understand about healthy eating, involve them. Learn together about good-tasting, healthy food and how to prepare it. Have them find things on their own that they want to try. Learn to cook together in fun cooperation. It is healthier than isolating yourself and feeling burdened by people who don't cooperate or understand. Young children need the life-skill building practice of learning to choose good vegetables and to wash and prepare them in healthy ways.

Make It Easy

It seems easier to reach into the refrigerator or cupboard and pull out a cookie or cake than take the time to fix a healthy meal. Have healthy food ready and easy to get to. Keep a bowl of fruit handy. Keep a container of cut vegetables within easy reach. Get and make healthy snacks ahead of time for when you know you will eat impulsively, and put them on the top shelf of the refrigerator and in the front of your cupboards. Get rid of unhealthful food in the refrigerator and cupboards.

Make It Healthy

Instead of hunching shoulders and rushing to get the cooking done, straighten, breathe, and use each stroke of washing and cutting as a relaxation or meditation. While standing to prepare food at the counter, don't slouch over the counter. Put your shoulders back with chin loosely in and your back held in neutral spine. Even if you need to hurry to prepare and cook, remember to be happy that you are fortunate enough to have things to prepare and cook. Don't ruin it with paying to put unhealthful food in your body.

Think Long Term

Food items are not worked off in single death bouts. Don't become discouraged if your body is not remade by the end of a week or a month. Small, daily calorie expenditures multiply over time. An easy 150-calorie-a-day walk translates into about 15 pounds a year. It works both ways—one extra 150-calorie-a-day piece of candy can mean you weigh 15 pounds more in one year. Think of the benefits of the walk plus not having the junk food. Make walking work for you with slow, steady reduction that does not tax your system. Slow weight loss is more likely to stay off, is easier on your heart, and spares bone and muscle.

Check for Extra Calories You Don't Need

For people who think they don't eat much and don't feel their weight reflects calories eaten, or think they don't eat unhealthy food, one way to check is keeping a list over a week or so:

- Count small amounts. You can cut many calories by not tasting foods as often when you cook, not licking icing from spoons, or not "just" breaking off halves of cookies to snack throughout the day. It can add up to hundreds of calories each day.
- Alcoholic drinks can add several hundred calories, plus hundreds more from bar snacks.
- Remember soda when you tally calories. Drinking soda is not healthy, whether diet brand or not. You don't need to harm your body in that way.
- Gum, mints, and small candies can have 10 to 15 calories each. It doesn't sound like much until you remember you eat a few dozen a day. Give some thought on why you have to keep your mouth moving so much of the time.
- Create more peace in your body. For better breath and stopping dry mouth, chew fresh green mint leaves or fennel seeds.
- Eighteen calories for a teaspoon of sugar doesn't sound like much until you count up all the two-packs in several coffees and teas a day. Milk, honey, and creamers add hundreds more.
- A big bag of chips, caramel corn, snack crackers, or cheese curls has over 1,000 calories, as does a can of roasted nuts. This amount accounts for more than half the calories most people need in a day.
- Trail mix and granolas are deliberately made to be high-calorie to sustain extended efforts in difficult terrain. They are not a low-calorie food or a food for daily life or regular snacks in a sedentary day. Half a cup of granola usually has over 200 calories. A big bowlful can have three to four times that. Adding milk or milk substitutes can add up to a 1,000-calorie snack. Many granolas are not healthful snacks; they contain refined flour and sugar. It is usually better to have fruit and nuts.

- Salad bars often have vegetables with large quantities of dressing and mayonnaise. Add cheese, croutons, nuts, olives, bacon bits, meats, and the like, and you can easily eat 3,000 calories in a single meal.
- Sport bars average 200 to 300 calories. They don't make you healthy or able to do sports just by eating them. Eating several is more than you need for exercise.
- Don't eat unhealthy foods thinking they are healthful for containing a little fruit or vegetables. Packaged fruit cups are full of sugar and syrup. French fries are not good for you, even though they are made from potatoes.
- Stop snacking while watching television.
- Sometimes, all it takes to lose the 10 or 20 pounds you want is to cut out one regular bedtime snack. Stopping just one 300- to 400-calorie-a-night snack will make a large difference.

Remember That "Diet Food" Is Food

Foods labeled as "diet food" are not magic potions that remove fat and calories from your body. They do not make you thinner by the action of eating them. They are food. Regular food. They have calories. Many have high sugar and fat content. They can make you fat if you eat too much of them.

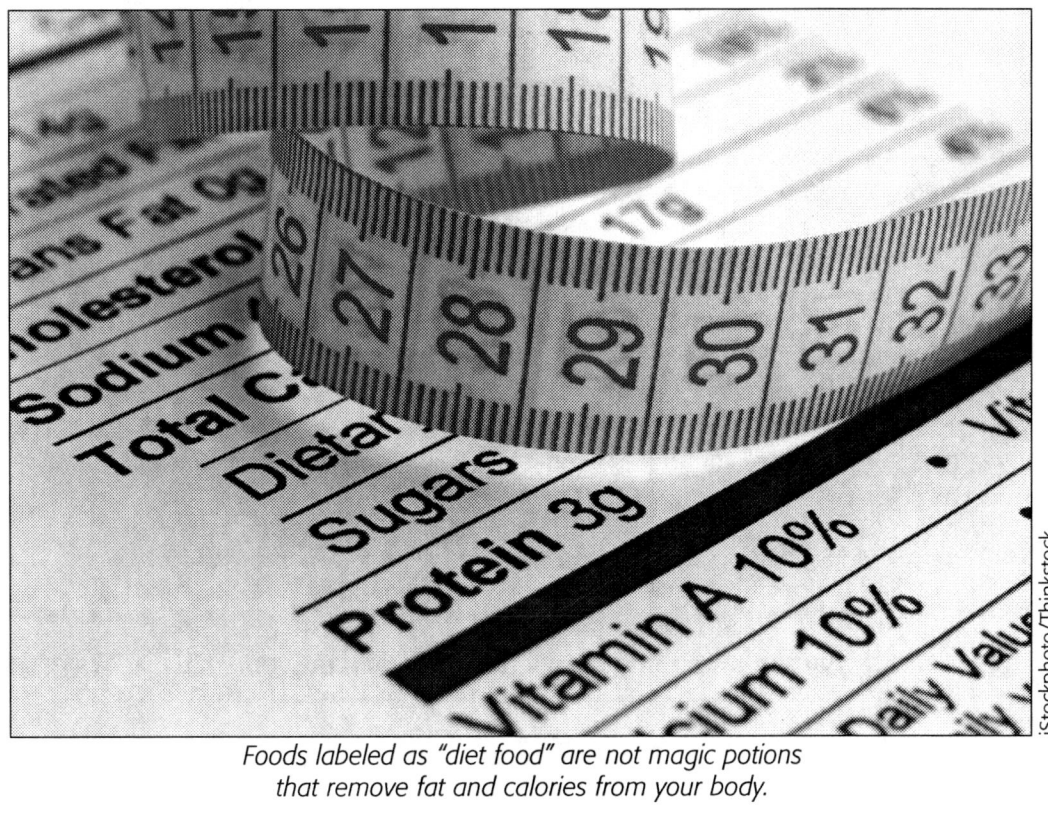

Foods labeled as "diet food" are not magic potions that remove fat and calories from your body.

What about meal replacement drinks? They also do not remove fat from your body just by drinking them. They are called "meal replacers" because you have one instead of anything else. You eat nothing else at all for that meal. Then, you don't snack or sneak food before the next meal. It is better to learn healthy eating habits. Have real meals that have fiber and all the combined nutritional components that can't come in a can. Use a meal replacer when you are rushing somewhere and are really missing a meal. Don't have it in addition to your other meals as a snack. The extra calories will store as fat.

Increase Physical Activity

A major factor in becoming overweight is a sedentary lifestyle. If you reduce activity enough to gain only one pound per year, think how much heavier you will be in 20 years. Think about only two pounds per year. You will probably not notice these gains on a day-to-day basis. Small things add up. Responsible plans for long-term weight loss include exercise. Exercise, in almost all cases, is a healthier, more effective weight-loss method than starving yourself. A University of California study found that most of those people able to remain slimmed down were those who started exercising regularly.

If you think that not having time to exercise is the problem, you have good news. Thinking that your life and your health are two separate things is the problem. You don't have to stop your life to get exercise.

Some people prefer organized exercise classes. They will drive to a gym and take the elevator to an exercise class, but hate to go out for a walk. They may not be getting the functional movement that develops their body in the way it needs for real-life movement. You do not need a gym or special clothes or equipment to get aerobic or weight-lifting exercise. It is more "natural," now called "functional" exercise, to get healthy exercise outside of a gym.

For both active and resistance exercise indoors and out, remember that daily healthful movement easily accumulates from your healthy bending, balancing while dressing, taking the stairs, and other daily, real-life movement. Find an activity you like anyway, such as going to a dance club, bicycling, or walking. Bend correctly for all the hundreds of times a day you need to bend. Make your life active. Try all kinds of things until you find something you love to do.

> The modern inactive life goes against developmental human history and the design of the human body to be active. Going to a gym today is only a substitute for a natural active life.

- See if you would like to commute by bicycle, where feasible, to work, or various errands. Grocery shop by bike, and use a backpack or bike baskets to carry home groceries. If not as much fits on the bike as the car, then you will spend less money and eat less. Maybe you will make more frequent trips by bike for more exercise.
- Improve your legs on the stairs instead of only waiting for escalators and elevators. You may beat the elevator.
- Go outdoors for a break every day that you can, for fresh air, sunshine, and fun movement. Instead of a smoking break, or a donut/Danish break, take a walk-and-stretch break, and have an orange and some raw almonds. Bend properly all day. You probably bend hundreds of times daily for the files, the trash can, to jot a message while standing, to pick up mail, or any number of other things. Bending over at the waist is terrible on your back. Use your legs, keep your torso upright, and burn calories with every bend. Get free bending and spiritual exercise by cleaning your closets to donate clothing and household items to give warmth and help someone in need.
- Have fun. Skate, bowl, cycle, walk, go dancing, work on your gardening, shoot hoops, take food to shut-ins and get them moving, too, with improvised exercise of moving arms and legs, clapping, singing, and having fun.

The human body was designed for activity and was active through the eons. In much of the "developing world" today, people commute by bicycle, regularly lift and carry loads, and sit and rise from the floor often. Modern life became inactive, bringing diseases of inactivity with it. Going to the gym is just a substitute (and often a poor one) for having an activity level that seems to be programmed into the human body for health. With practice, you can find activities that are fun and do them often until they become a natural, healthy part of your life.

Make It Fun

When you make a list of all the unhealthful food you eat, and how little you move as part of your real, daily lifestyle, weight gain is no longer a mystery to blame on metabolism or minor factors. Take a moment to breathe and think. Reflect on life as a brief gift, rather than something to harm through neglectful, undisciplined habits. Be excited about changing to good things. Don't just call it a diet to have to "stick to," but the way you want to live a quality life.

Eat healthfully and increase daily activity level by making common lifetime activities part of your exercise. Controlling weight without diets can become easy, safe, good feeling, and fun lifetime habits.

How to Control Your Weight

- *Reduce Fat and Refined Sugar.* You get too much fat and sugar in obvious ways, like fried food, rich desserts, and high-fat dairy products. You can also get too much fat and sugar in ways you don't always notice—in sauces, salads, packaged convenience food and snacks, and added to vegetables.
- *Make Your Own.* Homemade food is healthier and cheaper than convenience foods, and it can be quick and easy to make. It produces less litter, too.
- *Substitute.* Substitute good-tasting, healthy foods for unhealthy ones. Be creative, and find foods you like.
- *Eat Less Simple Sugar.* Stopping refined sugar and refined flour products is a factor in stopping food cravings.
- *Be Prepared.* Pack healthy food to take with you to places that have only unhealthy food.
- *Improve Your Mindset.* Check your ideas about what you think is healthful and why.
- *Make It Easy.* Have healthy food ready and easier to get to than junk food when you know you will eat impulsively.
- *Lose Real Fat Weight.* Rapid-loss fad diets concentrate on losing water and muscle. Steady weight loss with more movement and less bad food will reduce body fat weight, is easier on your heart and skin, and spares bone and muscle.
- *Check for Extra Calories You Don't Need.* Sometimes all it takes to lose the 10 or 20 pounds you want is to cut out idle snacking, foods that are terrible for you anyway, and late-night extra meals.
- *Remember That "Diet Food" Is Food.* It does not make you thinner by eating it. It makes you fat if you eat too much of it.
- *Increase Physical Activity.* A major factor in becoming overweight is a sedentary lifestyle.
- *Make It Fun.* Make your new, healthy lifestyle a fun one so you live it as a real life to enjoy, rather than making it something to do, and then stopping as soon as you can.
- *Eat More Slowly.* Put your fork or spoon down between bites. Breathe. Eat less.
- *Turn Off the Television.* Enjoy the quiet, or have a meaningful conversation with friends and loved ones over dinner.
- *Bend and Lift Properly.* Do you damage your back and knees all day, every day with bad, bent-over bending? Instead, you could burn hundreds of calories and exercise their legs by lifting with torso upright and knees bent. Examples include getting things out of the refrigerator, desks, low shelves, and closets; tying shoes; picking up mail, babies, papers, and laundry; vacuuming; making beds; leashing pets; and countless others.

Section Two

Exercise Nutrition— What You Need To Know

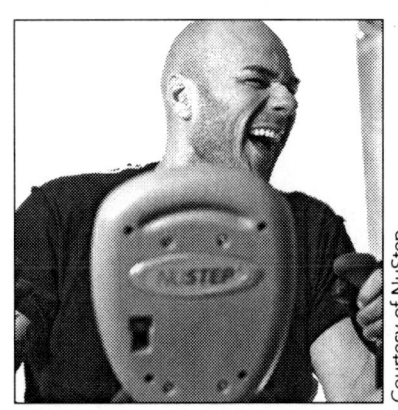

CHAPTER 3
CARBOHYDRATES

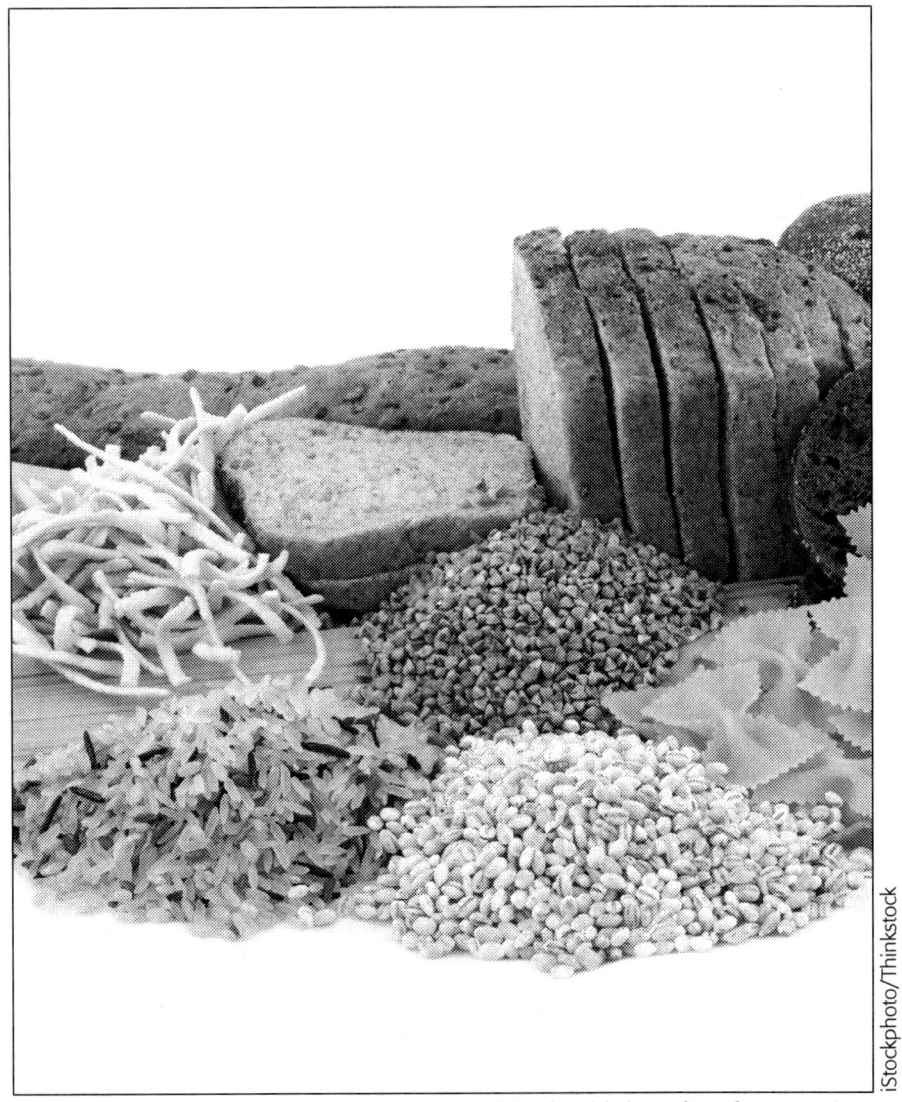

It is important that individuals are aware of the health benefits of consuming quality carbohydrates in quantities that support energy balance.

What Are Carbohydrates, and Why Do We Need Them?

The primary function of carbohydrates in humans is to fuel organ activity, particularly the brain, heart, and skeletal muscle. In fact, some carbohydrates may also play structural roles at the cellular level. In reality, however, carbohydrate's role as a fuel source is absolutely vital.

Carbohydrates contain the elements carbon, hydrogen, and oxygen and are classified according to size as monosaccharides, disaccharides, or polysaccharides. The smallest unit of a carbohydrate is called a monosaccharide and comes in one of three forms: glucose, fructose, and galactose. Glucose is often referred to as "blood sugar." Fructose, which is commonly found in fruit, is often referred to as "fruit sugar," while galactose typically exists in milk.

The next largest form of carbohydrate is called a disaccharide, a configuration that is simply the combination of two monosaccharides. The most common disaccharides in the human diet are sucrose, or "table sugar," lactose, or "milk sugar," and maltose. Sucrose molecules, which contain one fructose and one glucose molecule joined together, are abundant in the human diet. A lactose molecule combines a glucose molecule and a galactose molecule together. A maltose molecule connects two glucose molecules together.

The most complex form of carbohydrate is the polysaccharide, which involves a lengthy chain of monosaccharides joined together. Three of the most common polysaccharides are starch, fiber, and glycogen. Starch is the storage form of carbohydrate in plants, is abundant in the human diet, and is easily digested by the human body. Fiber also involves a chain of glucose molecules. Humans cannot break the bonds between these molecules, however, because they lack the appropriate enzymes to do so. As a result, fiber passes undigested through the gastrointestinal tract. Glycogen is the storage form of carbohydrate in animals and is found in both the liver and skeletal muscle. Unlike starch, which under a microscope looks fairly straight-chained, glycogen is highly branched. This attribute is physiologically beneficial because digestive enzymes work from the ends inward. Since glycogen has so many branches, the enzymes have a large surface area on which to work. As a result, glycogen can be broken down quite rapidly and digested by the human body.

Digestion and Metabolism of Carbohydrates

Carbohydrate digestion begins in the mouth with the aid of the enzyme salivary amylase. Salivary amylase starts digesting starch molecules by cleaving polysaccharide chains into smaller maltose molecules. Anyone who has placed a piece of bread in their mouth and noticed a sweet-like taste has experienced this process firsthand. Carbohydrate digestion in the mouth proceeds only to the level of the disaccharide. In fact, further digestion of disaccharides does not continue until they reach the small intestine. This situation exists because the acidic environment of the stomach interferes with the action of salivary amylase, an interplay that essentially stops digestion at this juncture.

In the small intestine, the remainder of any consumed starch molecules is acted upon by pancreatic amylase, which degrades any remaining polysaccharides into disaccharides. Even disaccharides are too large to cross the intestinal wall and must be further split into monosaccharides before being assimilated into the bloodstream. Sucrase, lactase, and maltase are enzymes located in the intestinal wall that split disaccharides into their respective monosaccharides. The resulting monosaccharides cross the intestinal wall and travel via the bloodstream to the liver, where fructose and galactose are converted to glucose. Eventually, all ingested carbohydrate ends up in the liver as glucose.

The ultimate fate of ingested glucose depends on the metabolic demands of the body that exist at the time of digestion. One consequence is that glucose will be used as fuel by active organs. In addition, glucose can be converted to glycogen in the liver and skeletal muscle if glycogen stores are depleted in these locations. It should be noted that the liver and muscle can only hold so much glycogen. Finally, if organs are fueled properly and glycogen stores are full, the third destination for the ingested carbohydrate is storage as fat. The liver can take the excess glucose molecules, convert them to fatty acids, and store them as triglycerides in adipose tissue. Any form of carbohydrate not used as fuel or stored as glycogen will end up as adipose tissue triglyceride. This situation does not mean that this carbohydrate will remain in adipose tissue forever.

Normally, blood glucose levels are carefully maintained at a prescribed level by various internal-control mechanisms. For example, when blood glucose levels begin to fall, the body will respond by breaking down glycogen and releasing glucose into the bloodstream. Similarly, when blood glucose levels rise, the pancreas will secrete the hormone insulin into the blood to trigger the uptake of glucose into cells, thereby reducing blood glucose down to normal levels.

Carbohydrates and Health

A popular myth exists that all carbohydrates are bad for health and that it is best to avoid these foods in the diet. What many people fail to realize is that carbohydrates come in different levels of quality. Poor-quality carbohydrates are made from processed, bleached flour. This type of carbohydrate usually lacks dietary fiber and may or may not lack other vitamins and minerals. Processed products are often "enriched," a term that refers to the fact that some of the nutrients lost while processing these items are added back before packaging. Products containing simple sugars have both carbohydrate and calories, but often lack other quality nutrients, such as fiber or vitamins and minerals.

High-quality carbohydrates, on the other hand, are generally found in unprocessed plants, legumes, and grains, items that contain abundant vitamins and minerals, as well as energy. High-quality carbohydrates also have a high level of indigestible dietary fiber, plant matter that helps keep the colon healthy and allows for stool to pass easily.

Plants also contain biologically active compounds called phytochemicals. Since phytochemicals are not required to sustain life, they are not nutrients. They are, however, believed to promote health and prevent disease. The scientific community has identified hundreds of phytochemicals, but their specific functions are not clear. While some data exists to support a relationship between the intake of phytochemicals and the prevention of disease, no established Dietary Reference Intakes (DRIs) have been identified for these compounds. One example of a phytochemical is lycopene, which is the compound that makes tomatoes red and watermelon pink. Scientists believe that a positive relationship exists between the intake of lycopene and a reduced risk of prostate cancer. It is unclear, however, how much of this substance is needed in the diet. Furthermore, many supplement manufacturers are now isolating lycopene, putting it in a pill, and using the limited scientific data to market the product for health promotion. One of the main problems with relying on supplemental forms of vitamins, minerals, and phytochemicals is that these compounds may not work the same way when they are isolated from other components that are normally found in whole foods. For example, the lycopene in tomatoes may interact with other antioxidant nutrients or unidentified phytochemicals to have the protective effect described previously.

Eliminating carbohydrate-rich foods from the diet means that antioxidant nutrients and phytochemicals may not be consumed in optimal amounts for health and disease prevention. As such, it is important that individuals are aware of the health benefits of consuming quality carbohydrates in quantities that support energy balance.

Relationship Between Fiber and Disease

Dietary fiber intake at appropriate levels may reduce the risk of certain diseases, such as colon cancer and diverticulosis. Diverticulosis is a medical condition that is common in older individuals and is characterized by pockets forming in the large intestine. These pockets generally develop after years of pressure from straining to defecate. With adequate fiber and fluid intake, stool passes easily and the risk of diverticulosis lessens. Diverticulitis occurs when diverticulosis pockets trap partially digested food and subsequently become infected and inflamed. This condition warrants the advice of a registered dietitian for treatment.

It is important to know that most Americans do not consume sufficient amounts of fiber in their diet. It should be noted that it is important to increase fiber intake gradually and to concurrently drink more fluids with enhanced fiber consumption; otherwise, constipation may result.

The DRI for dietary fiber in adult individuals up to 50 years of age is 38g per day for men and 25g per day for women. Reading food labels is a simple way to determine the fiber content of various food products. In this situation, individuals should search for the term "whole grain" and also look at the nutrition facts panel on the product.

Individuals should also compare whole grain versus white products. With minor changes, individuals can significantly add fiber to their diets while still eating their favorite foods. For example, whole-grain pasta can have 6g of fiber per serving versus one or less gram per serving in white pasta. Many cereals contain 10 to 15g of fiber in one half to one cup. On the other hand, individuals should not be fooled by the term "whole wheat." For example, whole-wheat products may be brown in color because the flour is not bleached, although these products may not have much more fiber than a white-flour product.

The Glycemic Index

Another myth that has gotten a great deal of publicity in recent years is one that states that foods with a high glycemic index (GI) are unhealthy because they cause a rapid rise in blood sugar after consumption. Many people associate an elevated level of blood glucose, regardless of how transient the rise, with diabetes, obesity, and heart disease. The problem with this line of thinking is that many factors can impact the measurement of a food's GI that have nothing to do with how healthy a food is, such as crushing or mashing, cooking, addition of acids, variety and origin of growth, maturation/ripening, and the addition of other nutrients, such as protein or fat.

GI is a precisely defined measurement that indicates how quickly blood sugar rises in a fasting person in response to the consumption of exactly 50g of available carbohydrate compared to a reference food, such as glucose or white bread. Foods are then loosely categorized as low, medium, or high, depending on how high blood sugar rises compared to the reference food. This measurement involves several limitations that make it unwise to use GI as a sole determinant of whether a food is unhealthy. One limitation is that the measurement is based on precisely 50g of available carbohydrate, instead of on a standard serving size. For example, carrots have a relatively high GI. In reality, however, virtually no one would eat the large quantity of carrots that are necessary to induce a rapid rise in blood sugar. Another limitation of GI is that it is based on single foods in isolation and ignores the impact that eating other foods simultaneously can have on GI. As such, not very many people eat plain pasta or a plain potato, both of which have a high GI. On the other hand, if butter, cheese, sour cream, or even broccoli is added to that potato, or the potato is eaten in a meal with chicken, for example, then the GI is reduced. If some sauce, chicken, vegetables, or meat are added to that pasta, the GI is further attenuated. A third limitation of GI is that great interindividual variability exists among people. For example, one person may develop hyperglycemia in response to orange juice, and yet not have the same response to pasta. In contrast, another individual may have the opposite reaction. Pasta causes that person to experience an increased level of blood glucose, while juice does not.

GI should be viewed as a tool and not a rule. For example, a marathon runner may want to eat a high-GI product, such as a sport drink, because that individual wants glucose to enter the bloodstream fairly rapidly to help spare glycogen during the activity, which lasts for several hours. On the other hand, foods should not be ruled out entirely simply because they have a high GI.

Carbohydrate Metabolism During Exercise

As discussed previously, the body can use carbohydrate, lipid, or protein for fuel during exercise. In a well-nourished state, protein contributes minimally as a fuel source (i.e., 5 percent of total). In reality, most of the fuel that the body needs comes from either carbohydrate or fat.

Exercise Intensity

Figure 3-1 shows that as exercise intensity increases, the body has a greater reliance on carbohydrate (CHO) for fuel. In Figure 3-1, exercise intensity is gauged in terms of METS, which is the maximum rate at which the body can consume oxygen during exercise. The greater the percentage of METS, the greater the level of exercise intensity.

Intensity (I)	Energy Source
I < 30%	Primarily fat
30% < I < 50%	Fat > CHO
50% < I < 70%	CHO > Fat
I > 70%	Primarily CHO

Figure 3-1. Energy source relative to the level of exercise intensity

As exercise intensity increases, adenosine triphosphate (ATP) demand increases. Which metabolic pathways can produce ATP quickly, with no need of oxygen to meet the elevated demand? One such pathway is the ATP-PC system. Because this system is very short-lasting, it is most relevant during explosive activities that last 10 seconds or less. The other system is glycolysis, which produces ATP at a relatively fast rate solely from the metabolism of carbohydrate. Viewing it from this perspective, it becomes apparent why carbohydrate is the primary source of fuel during high-intensity, short-term activities. Another reason that carbohydrates are used more readily than fats during high-intensity exercise is that an increased reliance on fast-twitch muscle fibers exists during such activity. These fibers have the essential machinery to support anaerobic glycolysis (i.e., more glycolytic enzymes and fewer mitochondrial and lipolytic enzymes). In addition, the hormonal profile observed during intense exercise—including increased levels of epinephrine, norepinephrine, and glucagon, and a decreased level of insulin—favors increased glycogen breakdown and glycolysis.

The problem with relying on glycolysis too heavily is that because it produces metabolic by-products that ultimately cause fatigue, glycolysis cannot continue indefinitely. Furthermore, since glycogen storage in the human body is limited, long-duration activities must have alternative fuel systems in order to continue unabated. Aerobic metabolism is a system that can continue for very long times with little accumulation of fatigue-inducing by-products. Immense quantities of ATP can be produced from the oxidation of fatty acids and to a lesser extent from the oxidation of glucose. Even though more ATP is generated from fatty acids in total, glucose breakdown provides more energy per liter of oxygen used. In an environment where oxygen is limited, such as during intense exercise, glucose is a more oxygen-efficient fuel. Oxidation of fat and carbohydrates to ATP is a relatively slow process that is not ideally suited for high-intensity activities. On the other hand, with appropriate training, the body's ability to oxidize substrates can be enhanced to enable an individual to work at higher intensity levels.

Fat Burning

One popularly held view asserts that exercising at a low level of intensity for a long duration is necessary to maximize fat burning. Although it is true that at low-intensity exercise a greater percentage of energy is derived from fat than from carbohydrates, the total amount of calories burned during such activities is relatively low. In fact, individuals would be far better off exercising at a higher intensity level because their total energy expenditure and fat burning would actually be higher than at lower intensities, even though the percentage of fat calories burned would be lower. However, the literature demonstrates as the intensity of exercise increases, so does the rate of injury, and most individuals do not maintain their exercise program at high intensities. For this reason, a balance of intensity and duration is optimal for long-term fitness.

To better understand the aforementioned point, it would be helpful to compare two 30-minute workouts—one at low intensity and one at moderate intensity. During the low-intensity workout, an individual would burn 200 calories, of which 80 percent, or 160 calories, would be derived from fat. During the moderate-intensity workout, an individual would burn 400 calories, but only 50 percent, or 200 calories, would be from fat. Although the percentage of fat burned during the moderate-intensity activity would be lower, the total number of fat calories used would be greater. This trend extrapolates to high-intensity exercise as well, with even more benefits. All factors considered, high-intensity exercise tends to enhance fitness improvements more so than low-intensity training. In addition, high-intensity exercise, because it also metabolizes carbohydrates, causes some glycogen depletion. As such, post-exercise meals containing carbohydrate should be consumed to replenish the body's glycogen stores before any carbohydrate gets converted to triglyceride.

Carbohydrate Needs

Sedentary But "Healthy" Individuals (With No Obvious Disease)

The adult DRI for carbohydrates is 45 to 65 percent of total daily calories. Expressing a person's daily carbohydrate needs numerically in the form of required carbohydrate calories that should be consumed may be somewhat confusing. Some individuals seem to prefer to have a carbohydrate target value expressed in grams. The following example illustrates the conversion of a 2,000 kcal per day diet that is 50 percent carbohydrate to daily carbohydrate grams:

- 2,000 x 50% = 1,000 carbohydrate kcal
- 1,000 kcal ÷ 4g/kcal = 250g of carbohydrate per day (a carbohydrate has 4 kcal per gram)

Although the carbohydrate range of 45 to 65 percent is relatively broad, it meets the needs of most healthy individuals. Some individuals may be more compliant and feel healthier at the lower end of the range, while other people may do better at the upper end. It is important to keep in mind that the DRI range only applies to healthy individuals. For example, for an individual with a disease or medical condition, the DRIs may not be appropriate. In such a situation, the individual should consult a registered dietitian.

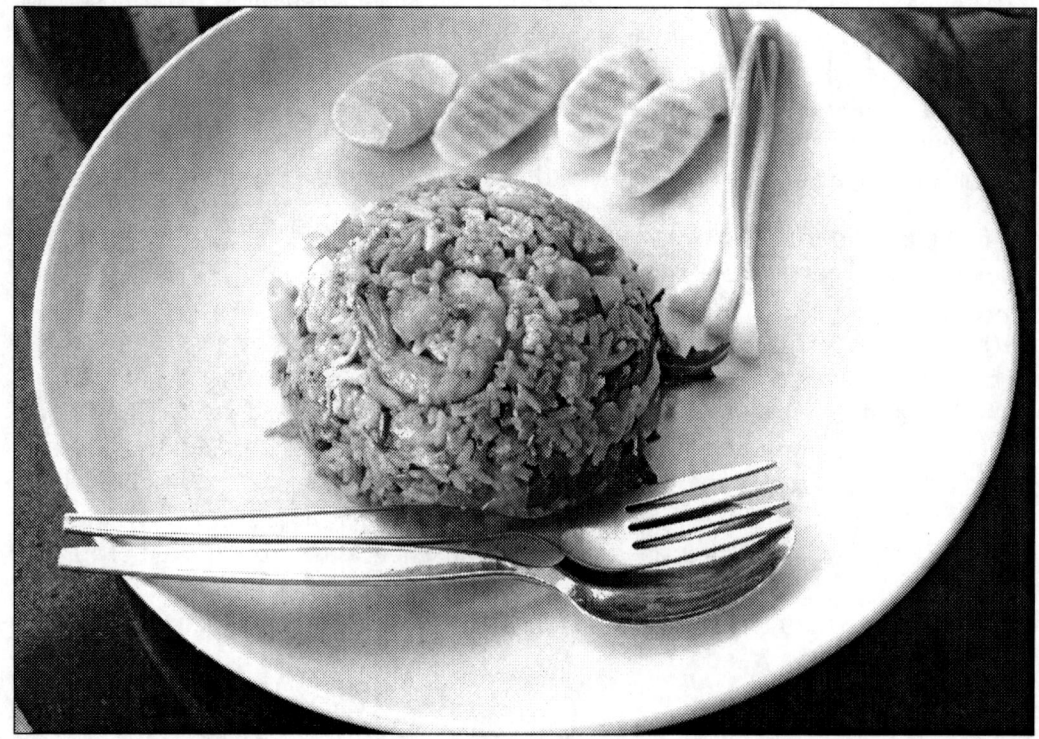

Although the carbohydrate range of 45 to 65 percent is relatively broad, it meets the needs of most healthy individuals.

Active, Healthy Individuals

Physically active individuals usually need more carbohydrate than their sedentary counterparts due to their increased use of glycogen as fuel. Because the DRI range for carbohydrates encompasses the increased need of active individuals, it is likely that such people would want to consume carbohydrate at the higher end of the DRI range. Finding the right amount of carbohydrate within the range to match activity levels is a trial-and-error process. Most competitive athletes engage in this undertaking and get to know what works best for them. On the other hand, many physically active individuals, college athletes, and recreational athletes need more guidance in this area. It should be noted that all of the aforementioned recommendations concerning carbohydrate consumption are for healthy individuals. People with a medical condition may need alternate guidelines.

The Importance of Carbohydrate to Performance

It is critically important to maintain glycogen stores during endurance activity. Once glycogen stores become depleted, the body will simply slow down, as fat becomes the predominant source of fuel. It is only during the later stages of prolonged exercise that protein may contribute up to 15 percent of the expended energy. Maximizing glycogen stores before activity and maintaining blood glucose during activity are paramount to being successful during endurance activities. The next three sections present strategies that can help individuals achieve these two objectives.

Before Exercise

No magical foods are needed for competition and sports; the issue is simply a matter of quantity and timing of eating. The underlying goal is to provide the body with glucose, without consuming so much food that it is uncomfortable or consuming so little food that hunger is triggered. Ideally, all carbohydrate consumed prior to exercise would be out of the stomach and in some stage of the absorptive process, whether it be circulating in the bloodstream, being taken up by cells, or crossing the intestinal wall. As the principles of digestion that were reviewed previously pointed out, liquids are digested faster than solids, and fiber slows the digestive process, which causes waste to remain in the colon longer. Although no DRIs exist for pre-exercise carbohydrate intake, most credible sources recommend 1 to 4.5g of carbohydrate per kilogram of body weight, depending on the type of food and the time of the event. Individuals who want more detailed meal-timing protocols should seek guidance from a credentialed dietetics professional.

People who consume carbohydrate before exercise are often preoccupied with GI. As such, they worry about reactive hypoglycemia, which is a transient condition where an individual's blood glucose level temporarily drops below normal in response to carbohydrate intake. While low blood glucose can certainly affect performance, this condition is not overly common. If a person suffers from this condition, however, lower GI foods or combinations of foods may be helpful. Any individuals who have this condition should work with a registered dietitian.

During Exercise

Ingesting carbohydrates during exercise does not enhance an individual's performance during all types of physical activity. In fact, only high-intensity activities lasting 30 minutes or more, or continuous endurance or intermittent high-intensity endurance activities lasting 60 to 90 minutes or more may benefit from carbohydrate supplementation during exercise. Credible sources recommend that consuming 15 to 20g of carbohydrate every 15 to 20 minutes is sufficient to meet the requirements of such activities. This amount translates to 1/2 to 3/4 cup of sport drink every 15 to 20 minutes. It is important to note that the aforementioned carbohydrate recommendation is merely a guideline and that, in fact, individual needs may vary. Some individuals may do better with 1/4 cup of carbohydrate supplementation during exercise, while others may prefer a full cup every 15 to 20 minutes. In reality, almost all elite competitors know the precise schedule of when they need to consume carbohydrate during exercise and what works best for them.

Recovery From Exercise

The major carbohydrate-related consideration for post-exercise, particularly if the activity was very long or intense, is to replenish glycogen stores. Glycogen stores can be replenished at approximately 5 to 7 percent per hour and can take 20 hours or longer to fully replete. Credible sources recommend that post-exercise intake equal 1.0 to 1.5g of carbohydrate per kilogram of body weight within 15 to 30 minutes after activity. It appears that the timing of consumption is critical and that the 30-minute deadline should not be extended. An additional 1.0 to 1.5g of carbohydrate per kilogram of body weight is recommended every two hours afterward, until a total of 7 to 10g per kilogram of body weight has been consumed. For example, the total post-exercise carbohydrate recommendation for an athlete who weighs 150 pounds (68 kg) is 476 to 680g (68 x 7 and 68 x 10). Accordingly, an amount equal to 68 to 102g carbohydrate should be eaten immediately after exercise and also at intervals two, four, six, eight, 10, and 12 hours post-exercise.

While this guideline is relatively simple, many factors are still being researched. For example, does the addition of protein to the carbohydrate further enhance glycogen resynthesis? In this regard, limited research exists to suggest that adding protein to carbohydrate during recovery enhances glycogen synthesis. More studies have been found that support the conclusion that carbohydrate intake is the important factor and that such consumption is independent of lipid or protein intake. It has been determined, however, that protein may play a significant role in post-exercise skeletal muscle protein synthesis.

Another controversial topic concerns GI. One of the traditional ways of thinking involved recommending high-GI foods post-exercise. While this conclusion is certainly not a bad idea, newer research suggests that total amount of carbohydrate is more important than the GI. As such, it is probably more practical to recommend that physically active individuals consume foods that are familiar to them and well-liked.

It should be kept in mind that the aforementioned recovery guidelines apply to athletes and physically active individuals who significantly deplete their glycogen stores. In fact, a person exercising for 30 minutes at a low level of intensity does not need to follow any of the aforementioned guidelines presented for before, during, or after exercise.

Carbohydrate Loading

Carbohydrate loading is a technique that typically begins a week before an endurance event, with the expressed purpose of maximizing glycogen stores. Research data suggest that when individuals deplete skeletal muscle and the liver of glycogen and then replenish, they can increase glycogen stores to two to three times their normal levels. The following four-point strategy is commonly used by athletes before an event. It is important to note that these are guidelines only and should not replace personalized strategies that have been developed by a credentialed dietetics professional:

- One week before an event, a long workout is performed, in an effort to deplete glycogen stores. For most people, depending on the intensity level of the session, this workout can take one to three hours.
- Moderate carbohydrate intake and a normal exercise routine are continued for the next three days.
- The routine is then reversed for the next three days. The carbohydrate intake level is high, and the exercise duration and intensity level is gradually tapered until the day before the event, which should be rest.
- On day eight, the day of the event, the individual's glycogen stores will hopefully be maximized.

How is it possible to tell if this process is working? In a research-laboratory setting, skeletal muscle biopsies can be performed to measure glycogen content. Obviously, this approach is certainly not practical. A simple alternative is for individuals to weigh themselves daily. For each gram of glycogen that is stored, almost 3g of water are stored with it. As glycogen is depleted in the first few days, body weight should decline; during the last few days during glycogen repletion, body weight should rise.

Carbohydrate Supplementation

Sport Drinks

A number of carbohydrate-supplementation products are on the market. As such, the sport drink is the "original" option in this regard, and one that remains very popular. Sport drinks generally contain approximately 14 to 15g of carbohydrate per cup. They also contain electrolytes that mimic quantities lost in sweat. Sport drinks are available in many flavors, a factor that serves to heighten their popularity. Research suggests that if a person likes the taste of a beverage, that individual will drink more. Specialty sport-drink formulas that contain extra electrolytes for people who are heavy sweaters are also available on the market, as are products with concentrated forms of carbohydrate that are designed for very long events.

Two questions concerning sport drinks that often come up are the following:

- *Why choose a sport drink over juice or soda?* The answer to this question is simple and based on scientific evidence. A 6- to 8-percent carbohydrate solution is best for the maximal absorption of glucose. In contrast, soda, juice, and fruit-flavored punches generally have twice the amount of carbohydrate per unit volume. This feature actually hinders glucose absorption and may cause gastrointestinal distress. In addition, sport drinks contain multiple forms of carbohydrate, including glucose, sucrose, fructose, and glucose polymers. Research suggests that this formulation is best for maximizing glucose absorption.
- *Can a homemade sport drink be made?* While the answer is "yes," some issues exist. For example, research suggests that fructose alone may cause gastrointestinal distress during exercise. A person could dilute juice with water (a 1:1 ratio) and then add a pinch of salt (many juices naturally contain potassium). The problem with this step is that the electrolyte levels of the beverage may be inexact, and the carbohydrate type may not be ideal. Unless individuals are adamant about making their own beverage, the commercially available formulas are quite inexpensive and readily available. Furthermore, they are even less expensive in the powdered form.

Another point that an individual who is training for an event and likes consuming sport drinks should consider is to find out what sport-drink product is being supplied, if any, during the event. This factor can be extremely important for a competitor who hates a popular flavor of a sport drink. As such, a person who has an aversion to a particular flavor will likely decrease intake of that sport drink, a step that could diminish that individual's level of performance.

Gels, Gummy Candies, and Other Products

In addition to sport drinks, a number of products—such as gels, jelly beans, and gummy candies—that contain both carbohydrate and electrolytes are available on the market. These products generally contain 25 to 30g of carbohydrate per packet. It is essential that individuals read these labels carefully, because some of these products may contain other unwanted ingredients, like caffeine or herbs. Among the benefits of these products is that they are small and portable. The primary thing that they lack is fluid. As such, it is still important to consume water if these products are taken before, during, or after exercise.

Bars

Quite a few bars exist on the market. Content-wise, they range from being high in carbohydrate to high in protein. Although the carbohydrate in these bars can fuel movement, these bars are not practical, because of the inconvenience and discomfort associated with chewing them. Furthermore, they contain no fluid.

Many bars are marketed as "energy bars." All too often, the term "energy" is abused on products. Given that a kilocalorie (kcal) is a unit of energy, anything that contains calories could be viewed as an "energy" food. Many products that use this term imply that their product is special or that the item may contain stimulants such as caffeine. Regrettably, no regulations currently exist on the use of this term on food product labels. For example, if a person is looking to ingest a snack of 25 to 30g of carbohydrate, does that individual need a specialized energy bar marketed for athletes or can that person get the same carbohydrate benefits from a common, inexpensive cereal bar? In reality, many of the "supermarket variety" bars use all-natural ingredients with no preservatives, and at a much lower cost than sport bars.

When looking for a high-quality bar, the most appropriate choice is one that contains at least 2g each of fiber and protein, has less than 1g of saturated/trans fat combined, and is made from whole grain. In fact, whole grain should be listed first on the ingredient's label. Individuals who are looking for bars that are relatively high in fiber have many options, including a number of bars that each contain more than 10g of fiber.

Summary

Glucose, the usable form of carbohydrate in the body, is an important fuel source for many organs, including skeletal muscle. A person's dietary carbohydrate needs will vary, depending on the level of physical activity. For athletes and physically active individuals, it is important to eat enough carbohydrate to sustain activity demands, and to take in additional carbohydrate before, during, and after exercise in order to maintain and replenish glycogen stores. Many food sources are rich in carbohydrate. In addition, several types of carbohydrate-containing products are available for use during athletic events.

CHAPTER 4
LIPIDS

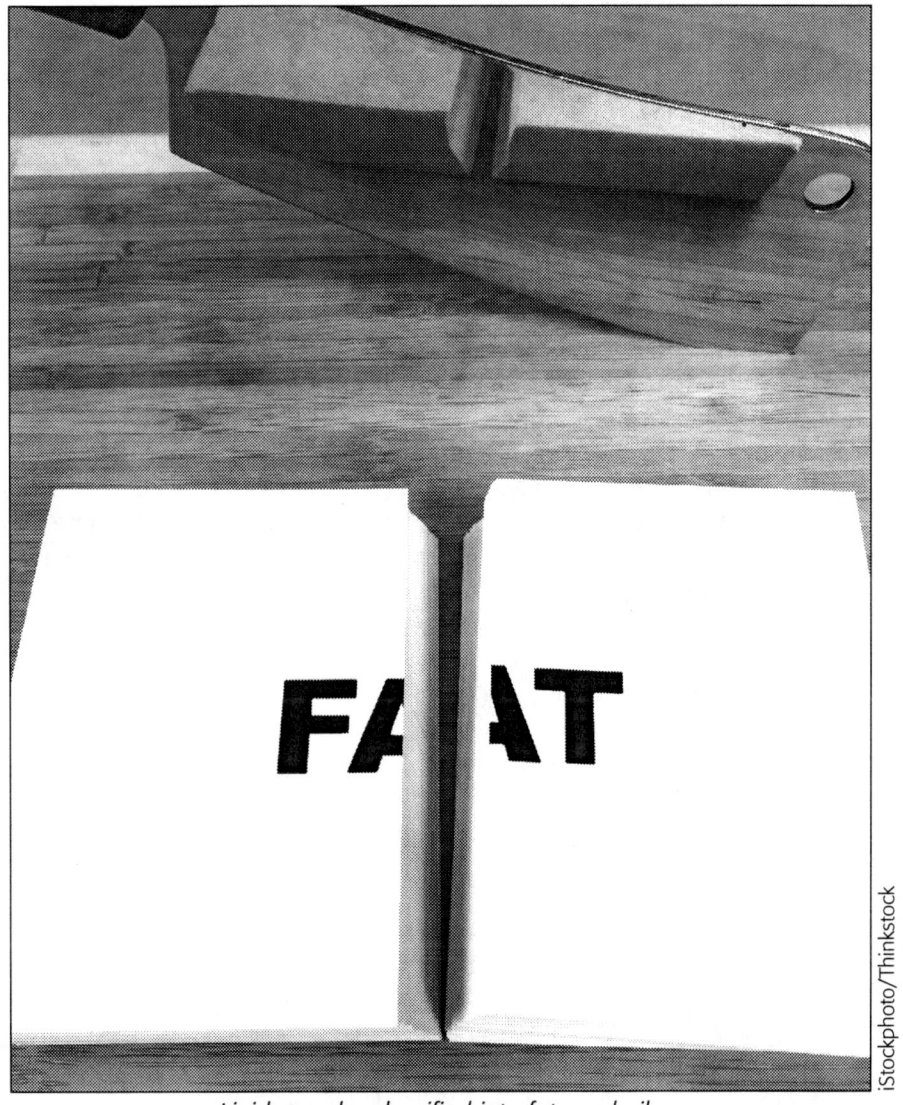

Lipids can be classified into fats and oils.

Lipids Defined

Lipids contain three elements: carbon, hydrogen, and oxygen. Each gram of lipid contains nine calories of energy. A primary function of lipids is fuel, but they are also helpful with insulation, protection, transportation, and adding flavor and texture to foods. The form of lipid most common in a Western diet and the variety stored in the human body is called a triglyceride (TG). A TG contains three fatty acids, which are composed of a long chain of carbon and hydrogen atoms bound together, connected to a small carbon containing molecule called glycerol.

Lipids can also be classified into fats and oils. Fats are usually solid at room temperature, while oils are liquids. Fats can be further classified by their degree of saturation. Saturated fats are those fats whose carbon atoms are bound to as many hydrogen atoms as chemically possible. Because saturated fatty acids are straight in shape, these molecules are tightly attracted to each other. It requires a lot of energy to separate them, which is why saturated fats tend to be solid at room temperature. Unsaturated fats, which include monounsaturated and polyunsaturated varieties, on the other hand, do not have the maximum number of hydrogen atoms attached to every carbon atom.

Whenever a hydrogen atom is missing, a double bond between two carbon atoms is in its place **(please don't stop reading; this is important, and it gets much more interesting soon).** Unsaturated fatty acids are not as strongly attracted to one another as are saturated fatty acids because every double bond creates a kink in the shape of the molecule. As a result, these fats tend to be liquid at room temperature. Monounsaturated fats—such as olive oil and canola oil—have only one double bond, while polyunsaturated fats—including most vegetable oils—have more than one double bond. Polyunsaturated fatty acids can be further categorized as either omega-6 or omega-3, depending on where the double bonds are located on the fatty acid. Both omega-6 and omega-3 fatty acids are essential, which means that they cannot be synthesized by the human body and must be consumed in the diet. Due to the high intake of fats in the Western diet, essential fatty acid deficiencies are not common. However, the ratio of these fatty acids in the typical diet is not ideal. Omega-6 fatty acids, which are found in many vegetable oils, are often consumed in abundance, while omega-3 fatty acids are more limited. Common sources of omega-3 fatty acids include fatty fish, flax seed, and certain nuts (e.g., walnuts and almonds).

Considerable attention has been given to the role of trans fatty acids in the development of abnormal blood lipids and heart disease. Trans fat is the common name for a type of unsaturated fat that has been shown to be decidedly unhealthy. For example, research has shown that trans fats raise "bad" (low-density lipoprotein, or LDL) cholesterol levels and lower "good" (high-density lipoprotein, or HDL) cholesterol levels. As such, consuming trans fats will increase an individual's risk of developing both heart disease and type 2 diabetes, as well as suffering a stroke.

Trans fats can be found in many foods, including stick margarines and shortenings used in baking and frying foods (e.g., lard). A number of years ago, lard (animal fat) was commonly used to bake and fry foods. A solid substance at room temperature, lard gives flavor to food and provides a desirable texture. Over time, it developed the reputation of being bad for health. While an individual who is attempting to bake something could replace the called-for amount of animal fat with vegetable oil, anyone who has ever tried to bake pie crust or chocolate chip cookies with vegetable oil knows that the taste and texture would just not be right.

Food manufacturers attempted to solve this problem by developing a vegetable-based product that tastes and behaves like animal fat, but without the unhealthy side effects, or so they believed. In fact, artificially adding hydrogen molecules to polyunsaturated vegetable oil does make them more "fat-like." They become solid at room temperature, prevent rancidity, and are ideal for baking and frying. The resultant problem, however, is that the hydrogenation process places hydrogen atoms on opposite sides of the double bonds, or in the "trans" location. Because trans fatty acids are straight—with no kinks—they resemble saturated fatty acids, even though they are still unsaturated. While this solid, vegetable-based compound has great cooking properties, it possesses the unhealthful side effects of saturated fats, such as elevated lipids and cholesterol, which results in a greater risk of heart disease.

Digestion and Metabolism of Lipids

The primary site of lipid digestion is within the small intestine. Lipids are digested best with the help of a compound called bile, which is an emulsifying compound made by the liver and stored in the gallbladder. The presence of fat in the small intestine stimulates the release of bile, which breaks the large lipid globules into smaller units, thereby increasing the surface area upon which lipolytic enzymes can act. Pancreatic lipase is the enzyme that breaks down TG into its component fatty acids and glycerol, which then cross the intestinal wall. Since lipids are not water soluble, they cannot travel in the bloodstream by themselves. Instead, they must be transported inside vehicles that are water soluble, namely lipoproteins.

Lipoproteins are predominantly lipid on the inside and protein on the outside. A chylomicron is a lipoprotein produced in the intestinal wall that carries absorbed dietary lipids and cholesterol through the lymphatic system to the bloodstream. The lipid located in chylomicrons has two fates. It is either delivered to active tissues and used as fuel or stored in adipose tissue as fat.

Most individuals who exercise have likely heard of HDL and LDL. These lipoproteins are produced when the liver converts excess dietary carbohydrate, lipids, and protein into lipoproteins and releases them into the bloodstream so that they can be used by body cells. The relative amount of lipid in the lipoprotein determines whether it is categorized as low or high density. Since lipid is less dense than protein, an LDL has more lipids than an HDL. Normally, LDLs are taken up by the liver and recycled back into the bloodstream as very low-density lipoproteins (VLDL), which target active cells and adipose tissue to unload their lipids. The uptake of LDL by the liver may be interfered with either by the consumption of saturated fat or trans fat or by the condition of obesity. Such interference contributes to elevated LDL levels in the blood. Over time, LDLs begin to degrade and release their lipids, including cholesterol, into the blood. Circulating cholesterol has been implicated as one of the major contributors to the development of arterial plaques and subsequent atherosclerosis. As a result, even though LDL is actually a lipoprotein, it is often called the "bad cholesterol" by the general public.

HDLs are important because these lipoproteins help to keep levels of total serum cholesterol within a normal range. HDL picks up cholesterol from arterial plaques and delivers it to tissues that can use it to make necessary compounds or send it back to the liver to make bile. This function is why HDL is often called the "good cholesterol," even though the characterization is not accurate.

Lipids and Health

The number-one cause of death in the United Sates is cardiovascular disease (CVD). Although CVD has a number of risk factors, two of the controllable ones are dietary intake and appropriate levels of physical activity. Because diets that are high in saturated and trans fats tend to increase levels of total and LDL cholesterol, they also elevate the risk of atherogenesis. One of the steps in the formation of atherogenic plaques is the oxidation of the LDL molecule. For health reasons, it is important to keep this oxidation under control. In that regard, it is believed that a diet rich in antioxidants and low in saturated and trans fats may be helpful. Antioxidant nutrients are abundant in fruits and vegetables and are present in whole grains. Unfortunately, taking antioxidants in a supplemental "pill" form may not have the same benefits. The full value and beneficial scope of antioxidants remains positive but factually cloudy, and more research is needed.

Some of the larger studies conducted do not necessarily support supplementation with antioxidants. Data from the Physicians' Health Study found no decrease in the risk of cancer, heart disease, or diabetes with 12 years of beta-carotene supplementation in 22,000 men. In the Heart Protection Study, 20,000 participants experienced no difference in heart attack rates after five years of supplementation with vitamin E, vitamin C, and beta-carotene (Heart Protection Study Collaborative Group, 2002). Data from the Women's Health Study indicate that taking vitamin E for 10 years had no effect in heart disease, stroke, or cancer rates for healthy female professionals. Conclusions from studies like these do not signify that antioxidants are unimportant for preventative health.

The relationship between dietary fat and cancer is not as clear as the relationship that dietary fat has with CVD. Despite the numerous studies published, no definitive answer exists. While a positive relationship may exist between cancer risk and consuming a diet high in fat and low in plant foods, the mechanisms of how fat consumption contributes to the development of cancer are unclear.

Omega-3 fatty acids are also believed to have an impact on health. In reality, the American diet is generally low in omega-3 fatty acids. This factor is particularly relevant when newer data that suggests that atherosclerosis and CVD are partially an inflammatory process is considered. Since omega-3 fatty acids may help control this inflammation, they may help prevent the development of both atherogenesis and CVD. Daily recommendations for the consumption of omega-3 fatty acids for optimal health are listed in the next section.

Dietary Needs

The DRI for total fat is 20 to 35 percent of total daily calories. Separate DRIs have been developed for omega-6 fatty acids and omega-3 fatty acids by gender and life stage. The adult DRI for omega-6 fatty acids and omega-3 fatty acids is 5 to 10 percent of daily energy needs and 0.6 to 1.2 percent of daily energy needs, respectively. Some individuals maintain a healthy lipid profile by adhering to the guidelines for the lower end of the total fat spectrum, while others fare better by following the suggested parameters for the higher end. It should be noted that people who select the upper end of the DRI range should be choosing healthy fats, not saturated or trans fats.

Quite a bit of data exists to support consuming a Mediterranean-style diet for maintaining optimal lipid profiles. While this diet is high in total fat, the fat intake tends to be primarily from healthy sources, such as fish and olive oil. The diet also includes fruits, vegetables, and whole grains. There is not a DRI for saturated or trans fats, since they are not required in the diet.

The DRI for lipids applies to both sedentary and physically active individuals. Competitive endurance athletes will often end up at the lower end of the range, due to their increased requirement for carbohydrate and protein. While research data are extremely limited, evidence exists to suggest that chronic intake of fat below 20 percent of total calories may result in a reduced level of testosterone production in men. It is important to keep in mind that these data cannot be used to draw an absolute conclusion. Furthermore, similar data in women have not been published.

Due to the considerable amount of information that exists regarding the health benefits of omega-3 fatty acids, a number people are turning to meals containing fish. The types of fish rich in omega-3 fatty acids include salmon, tuna, sardines, anchovies, striped bass, catfish, herring, mackerel, trout, halibut, mussels, crab, and shrimp. Since information on omega-3 fatty acids is not currently required to be noted on a food label, the most practical advice to give individuals who would like to eat more omega-3 fatty acids is to consume fish with darker flesh. Consuming too much fish, however, can lead to toxic metal poisoning, particularly mercury poisoning. The current recommendation for fish consumption is to limit it to 12 ounces per week.

Individuals who prefer an alternate source of omega-3 fatty acids have several options, including flaxseed, flaxseed oil, or nuts, particularly almonds and walnuts. If flaxseeds are to be consumed, they must be ground, since the whole seed is not digestible. In addition, the ground seeds should be kept in a freezer to preserve their freshness. Flaxseed and flaxseed oil often turn rancid very quickly.

Lipid Metabolism During Exercise

The TG stored in adipose tissue is a basic source of fuel during exercise. The other lipid storage compartment that plays a role in providing fuel during exercise is intra-muscular triglyceride (IMTG). As the intensity level of the exercise bout increases, the body relies more on IMTG to contribute to the total portion of the fuel that is supplied by fat. In fact, individuals who are trained have a larger reserve of IMTG than untrained individuals, which makes sense, because IMTG is more rapidly available due to its location than adipose tissue TG. The adipose tissue TG must be first broken down and transported to the skeletal muscle before it can be used. In addition to having a greater quantity of IMTG, a trained individual also has the ability to use more fat for fuel. As a result, this person can spare glycogen better than an untrained person.

Fat Loading and Performance

Since trained individuals can use more fat for fuel than untrained persons, the idea of increasing a person's consumption level of fat to improve their exercise performance level has been advanced in some quarters. In that regard, a few studies have examined the concept of employing fat-loading to enhance an individual's performance level during physical activity. The data, however, show that high-fat diets do not result in a performance benefit and, in fact, may be undesirable from a palatability and long-term health standpoint.

Summary

Several types of lipids exist in the diet, some of which are better for a person's health than others. While the body has minimal required levels of essential fatty acids, the overconsumption of other types of fatty acids can increase an individual's risk of developing cardiovascular disease. Fat is an important fuel source for the body, especially during low-intensity or prolonged exercise. While athletes tend to experience some metabolic adaptations to fat metabolism, the dietary recommendations for these individuals do not differ from the general population.

CHAPTER 5
PROTEINS

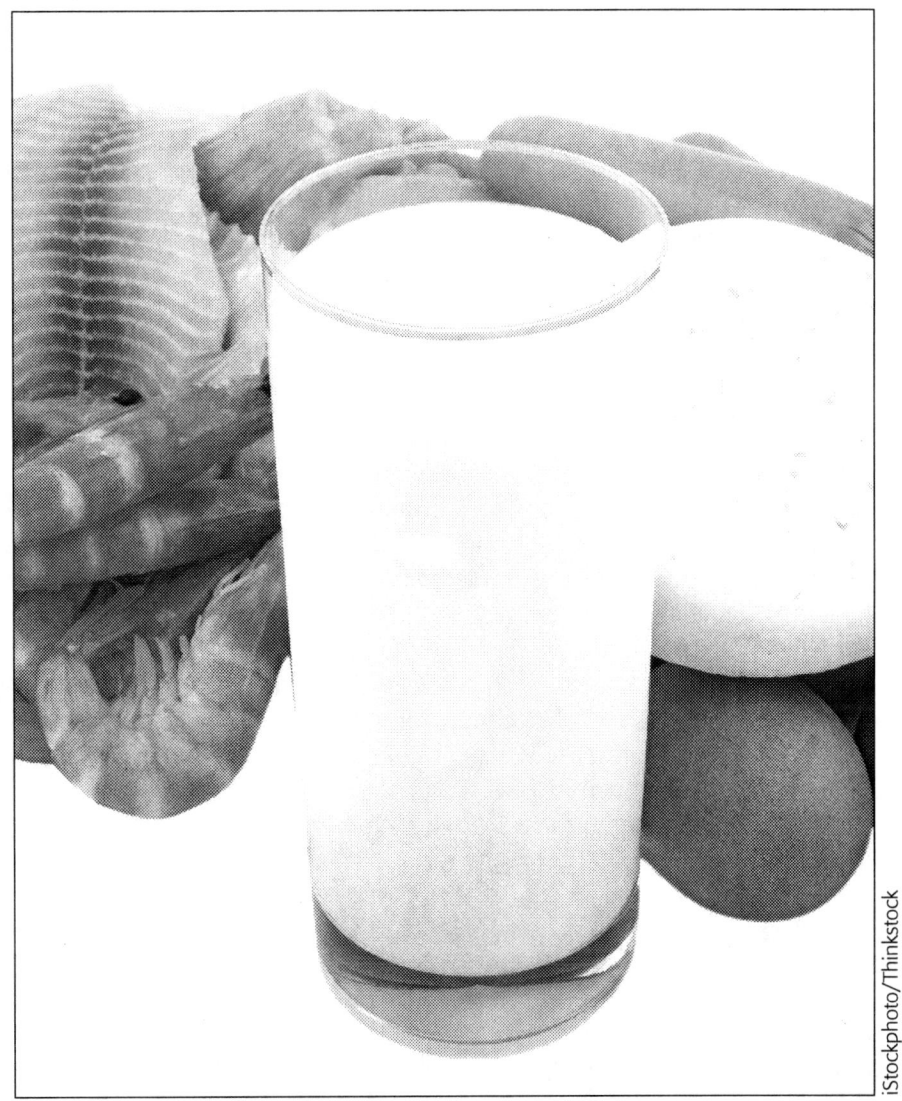

Daily protein needs are greater for active individuals and athletes than for sedentary individuals.

Protein Classification

Protein contains the following four elements: carbon, hydrogen, oxygen, and nitrogen. Protein has many functions and can be categorized as structural or regulatory. Examples of structural proteins include skin, cell membranes, and bone tissue. Regulatory proteins include enzymes, transport proteins (e.g., lipoproteins, hemoglobin), defense proteins (e.g., antibodies), contractile proteins (e.g., actin and myosin of skeletal muscle), hormones, protein pumps, and serum protein to help maintain fluid and electrolyte balance.

The smallest unit of a protein is called an amino acid. Two amino acids joined together form a dipeptide; three form a tripeptide; and many joined together form a polypeptide. One or more folded polypeptide chains form a protein molecule.

Protein Quality

Proteins in the human body are composed of 20 different amino acids. The nine essential amino acids (histidine, isoleucine, leucine, lysine, methionine, phenylalanine, threonine, tryptophan, and valine) are ones the body cannot make and are required in the diet. The 11 nonessential amino acids (alanine, arginine, asparagine, aspartic acid, cysteine, glutamic acid, glutamine, glycine, proline, serine, and tyrosine) can be synthesized in the body and, therefore, are not required in the diet.

Complete proteins contain all of the essential amino acids in one product, while incomplete proteins lack at least one. A good rule of thumb: if a product is animal flesh or comes from an animal, then it is a complete protein. Soy protein, from a plant, is one of the exceptions to the rule. Soy does contain all the essential amino acids, while most other plants lack at least one of the essential amino acids and are incomplete proteins. Vegans, who choose not to consume any animal products, may have concerns that their protein needs are not met. Many incomplete proteins, when combined together, provide all of the essential amino acids. For example, rice and beans or peanut butter and bread are great complementary proteins. It is important for vegans to have some variety in the diet if they are relying on complementary proteins, but protein needs can be met with careful planning. Vegans should also be mindful of the following nutrients: riboflavin, vitamin B12, calcium, vitamin D (if sun exposure is limited), iron, and zinc. These nutrients can be consumed in fortified foods or in a supplemental form if necessary.

Protein Digestibility-Corrected Amino Acid Score (PDCAAS)

The Protein Digestibility-Corrected Amino Acid Score (PDCAAS) is the Food and Drug Administration's official method for determining protein quality, accounting for both amino acid composition and digestibility. In general, protein from animal sources are more than 90 percent digestible; beans and legumes are approximately 80 percent digestible; and other grains and vegetables are less digestible overall but can range from 60 to 90 percent. The percent Daily Value (%DV) on a nutrition facts label may differ for the same quantity of different protein sources since the PDCAAS is used. For example, both 1 ounce of meat and one half cup of cooked beans contain approximately 7g of protein. However, the foods would contribute differently to total amino acid needs and, therefore, the %DV would be different on the label.

Biological Value

The term biological value (BV) is often used by supplement manufacturers to promote their product as being superior to another product or to foods. BV compares the amount of nitrogen absorbed from the diet to the amount retained in the body for maintenance and growth. Numeric values are available for many foods, but it is much more practical for a client to list or group those foods that have a high BV. For example, most animal foods have a similar value and are considered high BV protein sources.

Digestion and Metabolism of Protein

Protein digestion begins in the stomach with the aid of pepsin. However, the primary site of protein digestion is the small intestine, where enzymes called proteases digest the proteins into smaller units for absorption. Unlike dietary carbohydrates that must be broken down to the smallest unit (monosaccharides), proteins can be absorbed as tripeptides, dipeptides, and free amino acids. Each of these smaller units has its own transporter site to cross the intestinal wall, similar to having three different doorways for entry. Many supplement manufacturers claim that free amino acids are superior because they are already broken down from the joined amino acids. However, the small intestine is quite capable of absorbing the di- and tripeptides, as well as free amino acids. Additionally, supplemental free amino acids tend to be quite expensive when compared to the same quantity available in foods. Once the amino acids are absorbed, they travel to the liver via the hepatic portal vein.

When the amino acids resulting from protein digestion reach the liver, one of the following will occur:
- The nitrogen from the amino acids can be used to synthesize non-protein, nitrogenous compounds like creatine.
- The amino acids can be used to synthesize proteins.
- The amino acids can be used to synthesize nonessential amino acids.
- Some amino acids can be used to make glucose.
- The amino acids can be used for adenosine triphosphate (ATP) synthesis (under normal conditions, protein contributes approximately only 5 percent toward total energy needs).

If the prior needs are met, and extra amino acids are present, the liver can take the carbon skeleton from an amino acid, synthesize a fatty acid, and store it in the adipose tissue. When glucose or fatty acids are formed from carbon skeletons of the amino acid, or if the carbon skeleton is used for ATP synthesis, the nitrogen is removed, used to make urea by the liver, and then the urea is excreted by the kidney.

One of the metabolic fates of some amino acids is the ability to make glucose from glucogenic amino acids. The body will prioritize organ function, and the brain needs glucose to function. If a person is starving, glucose must always be maintained for the brain and can be made from the breakdown of skeletal muscle. One reason for the catabolism of skeletal muscle in individuals who are starving is that glucose cannot be made from a fatty acid (only a minimal amount can be made from the glycerol backbone of the triglyceride molecule).

Dietary fats have two fates: to be used for fuel or stored in adipose tissue (or intramuscular triglyceride). Glucose, from the ingestion of dietary carbohydrate, has three fates: to be used for fuel, stored as glycogen, or converted to fatty acids and stored in the adipose tissue. The body does not store protein as it does fats and carbohydrates; there is no equivalent to the glycogen stored in the muscle and liver or to the triglyceride stored in the adipose tissue. Skeletal muscle tissue is broken down in times of starvation but should not be considered the storage tank of smaller protein units or amino acids.

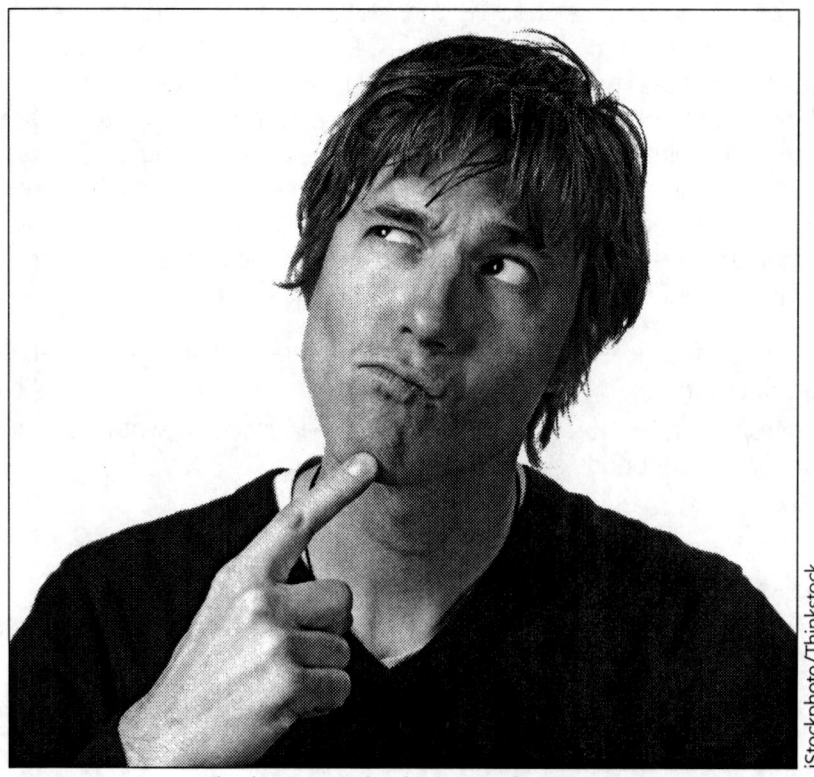

The brain needs glucose to function.

Dietary Needs

Dietary protein needs can be determined in the laboratory by a couple of methods. Measuring nitrogen balance is a classical method for precisely determining protein needs. Determining nitrogen needs is all that is required since protein is 16 percent nitrogen and is the only macronutrient that contains nitrogen. When the body is in negative nitrogen balance, it is in a catabolic state where amino acids are being oxidized. In contrast, when nitrogen balance is positive, the body is in an anabolic state, and amino acids are being incorporated into proteins. When the body is in nitrogen balance (nitrogen intake equals the nitrogen losses in the urine and feces), the protein requirements for the body are being met. This methodology requires that every drop of food intake be controlled and all excrements are collected. A sophisticated laboratory is needed where subjects reside in the facility and extensive equipment is available to analyze the nitrogen content of the food and bodily excretions.

Another newer method involves the use of radioisotopes to measure skeletal muscle protein synthesis and breakdown. With this methodology, the carbon molecules in an amino acid (most commonly leucine) are labeled or tagged with radiation to be traced through metabolic processes in the body. The amount of protein that is needed to reach a plateau in skeletal muscle protein synthesis is considered the protein requirement for the body.

Sedentary But "Healthy" Individuals (With No Obvious Disease)

The DRI for daily dietary protein in adults 19 to 50 years old is 10 to 35 percent of total calories or 0.8 grams per kilogram (g/kg) of body weight.

Physically Active Individuals and Athletes

Protein requirements are different for highly active individuals, as the DRI of 0.8g/kg will likely not be enough to maintain nitrogen balance. Based on the current available research data, endurance athletes need between 1.1 and 1.5g/kg per day, and resistance-trained athletes need between 1.5 and 2.0g/kg per day. The increased protein needs can be met with food, with no need for supplementation. Though many active individuals and athletes know they need more protein than their sedentary counterparts, some may consume several grams per kilogram of body weight per day. Can the body use all of this protein? The answer appears to be no. Studies measuring skeletal muscle protein synthesis find that protein synthesis plateaus at a protein intake of 2.0 to 2.4g/kg, meaning that protein intakes higher than this value are not being used to build muscle.

Protein Metabolism During Exercise

As mentioned in previous chapters, most of the fuel used during exercise comes from a combination of carbohydrate and fat, while only about 5 percent of the generated ATP (energy) comes from protein. An exception to this rule is at the later stages of prolonged endurance exercise, where protein can contribute up to 15 percent toward ATP production. The physiological explanation for this is simple: blood glucose must be maintained. As glycogen stores are depleted, blood glucose levels are in jeopardy. Since the body cannot make glucose from a fatty acid molecule, it must turn to protein for the synthesis of glucose.

Resistance training also results in a metabolic change in protein metabolism. During a resistance-training session, protein breakdown is generally occurring. Post-exercise, a marked increase in protein synthesis occurs such that the net protein balance is positive, which is necessary to build skeletal muscle. In order to promote this positive protein synthesis, adequate levels of both energy and protein need to be consumed. A question that remains to be answered is when this increase in protein synthesis is seen post-exercise. Unfortunately, the data are very limited because the methodology for determining protein balance is fairly new, quite expensive, and few laboratories have the ability to perform this research. At this point, the data suggest that increased protein synthesis occurs anywhere between immediately after exercise and up to 48 hours post-exercise. As research progresses, hopefully a more concrete answer will become available to establish more detailed protein-consumption guidelines.

Protein Intake and Supplementation

Types of Protein Supplements

One of the most popular forms of supplemental protein is whey protein. When milk curdles, the solid curds contain the protein casein, while the liquid portion contains the protein whey. Whey contains a high concentration of branched-chain amino acids (isoleucine, leucine, and valine), which play an important role in exercise metabolism and protein synthesis. Supplemental whey protein comes in different varieties:

- Whey protein concentrates can range in protein content, but generally contain approximately 80 percent amino acids. They also contain lactose, fat, and minerals.
- Whey protein isolates are the purest form of whey protein and usually contain 90 to 95 percent amino acids with little or no lactose and fat. They tend to be more expensive than whey protein concentrates.
- Hydrolyzed whey protein is broken down to peptides and, therefore, may reduce the potential for an allergic reaction in individuals sensitive to milk protein. It is commonly used in infant formulas and some sport drinks.

Another type of protein supplement is soy protein, which tends to be more commonly used by women. Soy protein supplementation should be considered with caution in some situations. This high-quality plant protein contains isoflavones, or plant forms of estrogens. Many breast tumors appear to be sensitive to estrogen and will grow when exposed to this hormone. The research data on soy consumption and breast cancer is unclear. Some studies suggest that the phytoestrogens in soy may bind to breast tumors and prevent endogenous estrogen from binding, thereby reducing the risk of tumor growth. Other studies suggest that the phytoestrogens in soy may bind to a breast tumor, behave like estrogen, and promote tumor growth. Until research data on this topic are clearer, it is best not to excessively supplement with soy if the person has a strong family history of breast cancer or if the disease is present. This does not mean all soy foods should be avoided, but people should not consume them in excess, especially in the supplemental form.

Strong data exists to suggest a relationship between soy protein intake and cardiovascular disease (CVD) and, in fact, the FDA has approved a health claim for this relationship. The data suggest that *replacing* 25g per day of animal protein with soy protein may reduce the risk of CVD. This statement appears on the label of food products containing soy. Notice the statement says to *replace* the animal protein with soy protein. This statement does not mean an individual should continue to consume a diet high in saturated and trans fats and then supplement with soy to get the protective effects.

Many male bodybuilders will avoid soy protein because of the fear of the phytoestrogens and the potential side effects, such as growth of breast tissue. Only one study in this area has been published, and it reported that 12 weeks of soy consumption in men did not reduce testosterone levels or inhibit lean body mass changes. More data are needed to confirm these findings, but consuming soy in modest amounts will likely not be problematic in altering hormone production.

Before and During Exercise

Based on the abundant research data, supplementing with carbohydrate before, during, and after exercise improves endurance performance. Since resistance training causes a disruption in protein balance, with a goal of increasing muscle growth, does supplementation with protein aid in this process? Unfortunately, not nearly as much research data is available examining this question as is available investigating carbohydrate intake. However, the available data can be reviewed to make the best of an athlete's training.

It appears that when carbohydrate alone or in combination with protein is ingested post-exercise, an insulin response occurs. Insulin is an anabolic hormone that plays a role in protein synthesis. It is not clear if carbohydrate and protein intake should be staggered or combined for maximal skeletal muscle protein synthesis. More research is needed on this topic.

Strong evidence exists for the daily protein needs to maintain nitrogen balance in various endurance and resistance-trained athletes. This question remains: how is the protein intake distributed over the day to maximize protein synthesis? Is it better to spread protein throughout the day or eat larger meals? Only a couple of studies have examined spaced versus single-dose protein feeding in older and younger women, and with conflicting results. Furthermore, these studies did not compare pre- versus post-training, and the results cannot be used to make absolute conclusions.

Many of the earlier studies on protein supplementation specifically examined the effect of protein intake post-exercise on skeletal muscle protein synthesis. Though studies are limited, it has been suggested that as little as 6g of protein ingested an hour or two post-exercise enhances protein synthesis, compared to no protein intake after the workout. More studies are needed before concrete conclusions can be made, but based on the available evidence, it would be wise to eat protein-rich foods post-exercise.

What about pre-exercise protein consumption? Even fewer research studies examine this question. A couple of studies came to the same conclusion: as little as 6 to 10g of protein ingested before a resistance-training workout resulted in greater protein synthesis compared to protein ingested post-exercise. Other studies found no difference in protein synthesis when protein was consumed before versus after exercise. From a physiological standpoint, this seems logical. It takes a few hours or more to digest food, depending on the meal size and nutrient composition. If protein synthesis increases post-exercise, having some amino acids readily available for the process will optimize the outcome. More data are needed before concrete recommendations can be made. However, it cannot hurt to consume a protein-rich snack prior to a resistance-training workout. For example, 6 to 10g of protein can be found in a yogurt, an ounce of meat or cheese, or a glass of milk.

Another common question: what is the best form of protein to maximize skeletal muscle protein synthesis? This question does not have a clear answer. While a few studies have been done on this topic, the answer is not conclusive. A recent study examined the effects of whey protein versus casein on body composition in recreational bodybuilders. This study did suggest that whey protein was better for reducing fat mass and increasing strength; however, this is only one study. More research of this nature needs to be completed before any conclusions can be made. Two other recently published studies examined the effects of milk versus soy supplementation during a period of resistance training. The results of both studies suggest that milk protein was superior; one study reported increased skeletal muscle hypertrophy, while the other reported a greater fat-mass loss. Though more research is needed, it is encouraging to see research supporting the consumption of a simple, inexpensive, and readily available product such as milk.

What is the optimal amount of protein in a single dose? This question may seem simple, yet few studies have been conducted examining this issue. An earlier study showed that larger amounts of protein (i.e., 40g) taken post-exercise may exceed the maximal effective dose. A more recent study examined doses of 0, 5, 10, 20, and 40g of protein and reported that 20g of egg protein isolate was the maximal dose to stimulate skeletal muscle protein synthesis without drastically increasing amino acid oxidation (an indication that the protein is being wasted).

Recovery From Exercise

Much research data support the use of carbohydrate intake post-exercise to replenish glycogen stores. In general, the research data do not support the need for protein ingestion post-exercise in order to maximize glycogen replenishment. However, protein intake post-exercise may play a significant role in maximizing skeletal muscle protein synthesis, and small quantities are likely to be effective. From this standpoint, it is probably a good idea to include some protein in the post-workout meal. The common recommended ratio of carbohydrate:protein is 4:1. Specialized products are on the market that have this perfect ratio in one product, but keep in mind that the post-exercise meal can be in the form of food. Research supports the fact that a glass of chocolate milk is an excellent recovery beverage. Many protein supplement powders promote their isoleucine and leucine content (both are branched-chain amino acids that play a role in protein synthesis). A 16-ounce glass of chocolate milk, 6 ounces of canned tuna, or one cup of cottage cheese has similar amounts of these "recovery" amino acids. In addition, the cost per gram of protein is much less with the food products than with the supplement. The supplement, however, does offer the convenience of being portable with no refrigeration required.

Summary

Protein has several functions in the body. Protein quality varies from different food sources, with the highest quality generally coming from animal products. Daily protein needs are greater for active individuals and athletes than for sedentary individuals; however, these increased needs can be met with food. While these daily protein needs are based on solid research data, there is not an abundant amount of research available to provide specific guidelines for protein intake before, during, or after resistance training to optimize protein synthesis. Limited data do suggest that small amounts of protein consumed before and after a resistance-training workout may be beneficial for maximizing skeletal muscle protein synthesis.

CHAPTER 6
VITAMINS AND MINERALS

Many vitamins play an important role in the energy systems. True vitamin deficiency may result in impaired energy metabolism and, hence, impaired performance.

Vitamins and minerals that are needed in the body in small quantities are classified as micronutrients. Vitamins can also be classified as fat-soluble or water-soluble. The fat-soluble vitamins—Vitamins A, D, E, and K—require dietary fat for absorption and are stored in adipose tissue. Water-soluble vitamins are not stored in the body, are depleted more rapidly, and, therefore, need to be consumed regularly. A common myth is that no toxic effects can occur from water-soluble vitamins since they are excreted rather than stored. While some water-soluble vitamins are not toxic, others are. The vitamins that have an established Tolerable Upper Intake Level (UL) have potential side effects.

Though each micronutrient has a specific function, some act as coenzymes in metabolic reactions. Despite a popular belief that vitamins provide "energy," they are not energy nutrients, as they do not contain calories. Many vitamins play an important role in the energy systems, but taking quantities in excess of physiological needs will not increase ATP production. However, true vitamin deficiency may result in impaired energy metabolism and, hence, impaired performance.

Dietary Reference Intakes

The Dietary Reference Intakes (DRIs) are published by the National Academy of Sciences (www.nationalacademies.org). The reports can also be accessed via the USDA website (www.usda.gov).

The DRIs are guidelines designed to be used as goals for almost all healthy individuals. For those who are free from disease and other medical conditions, the DRIs can be used as a goal for individual intake. The DRIs, categorized by gender and life stages, are quite easy to use.

However, in the DRIs, no category exists for athletes. Though research data on micronutrient requirements for athletes are not as abundant as for the general population, it appears that most of the DRIs are appropriate for healthy athletes and healthy active individuals. A few of the micronutrients may be of concern for athletes and are discussed in the following sections. For those who have a disease or medical condition, the DRIs should not be presented as a guide, and a registered dietitian should be consulted.

Vitamin and Mineral Supplements

Should you take a multivitamin/mineral (MVM) supplement or individual micronutrient supplements? Some people may believe that adding a MVM is a helpful "insurance policy" that cannot be harmful. Can the claims and ingredient quantities listed on the label be believed? It is questionable if 500 percent or 1,000 percent of the Daily Value (DV) is needed for the body. Greater than 100 percent of the DV may be toxic, so individuals should refer to the UL table of the DRIs. It is important to keep in mind that people may be consuming a MVM in addition to fortified energy bars, vitamin waters, fitness waters, and fortified foods such as soy milk or orange juice. A formal nutrition assessment performed by a registered dietitian may be warranted for those who use these products regularly.

Food should be the only source of these nutrients. For those nutrients that do have a UL listed, it can be very difficult to reach that level solely with food intake. It is the excessive nutrient intake from supplements and fortified foods that may cause problems.

If an individual eats well, but chooses to take a MVM to ensure nutrient adequacy, a product with no nutrients listed at more than 100 percent of the DV should be chosen. Even if someone does eat well and consumes 100 percent of the DV, they are unlikely to approach the UL. Some nutrients, for example calcium, may be listed on the supplement's label at lower than 100 percent of the DV because if each serving contained the full amount, the tablet would be too large to ingest. A DV lower than 100 percent does not imply that the supplement is inadequate.

Vitamins and Minerals That May Need Attention in Athletes

B Vitamins

Some data suggest that thiamin needs may be slightly greater in athletes. Thiamin is abundant in foods made with flour, corn, and whole-grain breads and cereals and is also available in many processed food products that have been enriched. Since most athletes and active individuals need more calories than sedentary individuals, the slightly greater thiamin need can be met by the increased food intake that is required to meet the demands of activity.

Antioxidants

A topic currently being researched is the role of antioxidants in the athlete's diet, especially the relationship between these compounds and muscle damage and soreness. The key antioxidant nutrients are Vitamin A (beta-carotene), Vitamin C, Vitamin E, copper, and selenium. At this time, data are controversial; some studies suggest an increased need for antioxidant nutrients with training, while others do not. Similarly, some report less muscle soreness with supplementation of antioxidants, while others do not.

Currently, the data do not support regular supplementation with antioxidant nutrients. Most of the long-term studies examining antioxidants and health focus on cardiovascular disease (CVD). These long-term studies report that antioxidant supplementation is not especially protective against CVD; other lifestyle factors must be studied and considered. However, consuming foods rich in antioxidants (e.g. fruits, vegetables, whole grains, and others, as shown in Figure 6-1) is likely beneficial for better health in all individuals.

Nutrient	Source
Vitamin A (beta-carotene)	Carrot
	Cantaloupe
	Papaya
	Mango
	Egg yolk
Vitamin C	Citrus fruits
	Peppers
	Strawberries
	Kiwi
Vitamin E	Nuts
	Seeds
	Avocados
	Canola oil
	Olive oil
Copper	Salmon
	Sunflower seeds
Selenium	Brazil nuts
	Tofu
	Tuna
	Mushrooms

Figure 6-1. Common antioxidant-rich foods

Calcium and Vitamin D

Other nutrients of concern—especially in young, female athletes—are calcium and Vitamin D, which are necessary for bone health. If an athlete has sun exposure and drinks milk, the Vitamin D intake may be adequate. However, young adult women need 1,000mg per day of calcium, and this need may not be met adequately in the diet alone. While it is possible to have enough calcium in the diet, usually three to five servings of dairy or calcium-fortified products daily are needed to fulfill the 1,000mg requirement. Some young women may avoid dairy foods because of the misconception that these are "fattening" foods. Nonfat milk and dairy products are good sources of quality protein and calcium despite the removal of the fat.

Phytochemicals and Health

Phytochemicals, while not classified as nutrients, are biologically active compounds that may reduce the risk of certain diseases like heart disease and cancer. Phytochemicals are abundant in whole grains, fruits, and vegetables. While databases are available to find the vitamin or mineral content of a food, the exact quantities of phytochemicals in foods are not readily available. Likewise, at this time, no DRIs or other specific recommendations for daily intakes of phytochemicals exist. The best advice for individuals concerned about meeting "daily phytochemical needs" is to consume a diet rich in whole grains that includes 8 to 10 servings per day of fruits and vegetables. Another common recommendation is to eat from the rainbow—to eat as many different colors of fruits and vegetables as possible. The vibrant colors of these plants are, in part, due to the phytochemicals found in them.

Some people may find this recommendation difficult to achieve. Knowledge of food portions will be helpful for clarifying serving size: a serving of fruit is approximately one half cup of juice or a piece of fruit the size of a tennis ball and a serving of vegetables is just one half cup of cooked or one cup of uncooked leafy greens. It can be challenging for people who currently eat no fruits and vegetables to increase their consumption level to 8 to 10 servings a day. It is best to set smaller, achievable goals. For example, a fruit smoothie or vegetables as a pizza topping contribute to meeting the goal. Another misconception: only fresh fruits and vegetables contain adequate nutrients. Generally, fruits and vegetables reach their peak nutrient content at their peak ripeness. It can be inconvenient to have to go to the market regularly to purchase produce, and fresh produce seems to spoil very quickly, especially when bought at the perfectly ripe state. Frozen fruits and vegetables are picked and frozen at peak ripeness and immediately packaged. Keeping frozen fruits and vegetables on hand can make it very convenient to incorporate these into the diet by adding frozen berries to a fruit smoothie, yogurt, or slice of angel food cake, or including frozen vegetables in a stir fry, as a pizza topping, or as a side dish.

What about taking a supplement containing phytochemicals instead of eating fruits and vegetables? Research in this area is new, without adequate data to establish firm recommendations. The bottom line is that it is not known if taking a phytochemical isolated in pill form will have the same effect as consuming the whole foods that naturally contain them. It could be that the phytochemical in question interacts with other unidentified phytochemicals or antioxidants present in the whole food and, when extracted, would not have the same beneficial effect.

Summary

Dietary Reference Intakes (DRIs) are designed to meet the needs of approximately 97 to 98 percent of the healthy population. These values are appropriate for individual use by those who are free of disease or other medical conditions. Athletes and highly active individuals may have slightly higher needs for a few micronutrients. However, these higher micronutrient needs can be met with the increased energy, or calories, required for training. Some nutrients warrant further consideration in athletes and active persons, and while supplementation of these micronutrients may be beneficial, care should be taken. For overall good health, it is prudent to use whole foods to meet the optimal intakes of micronutrients (including antioxidants) and phytochemicals.

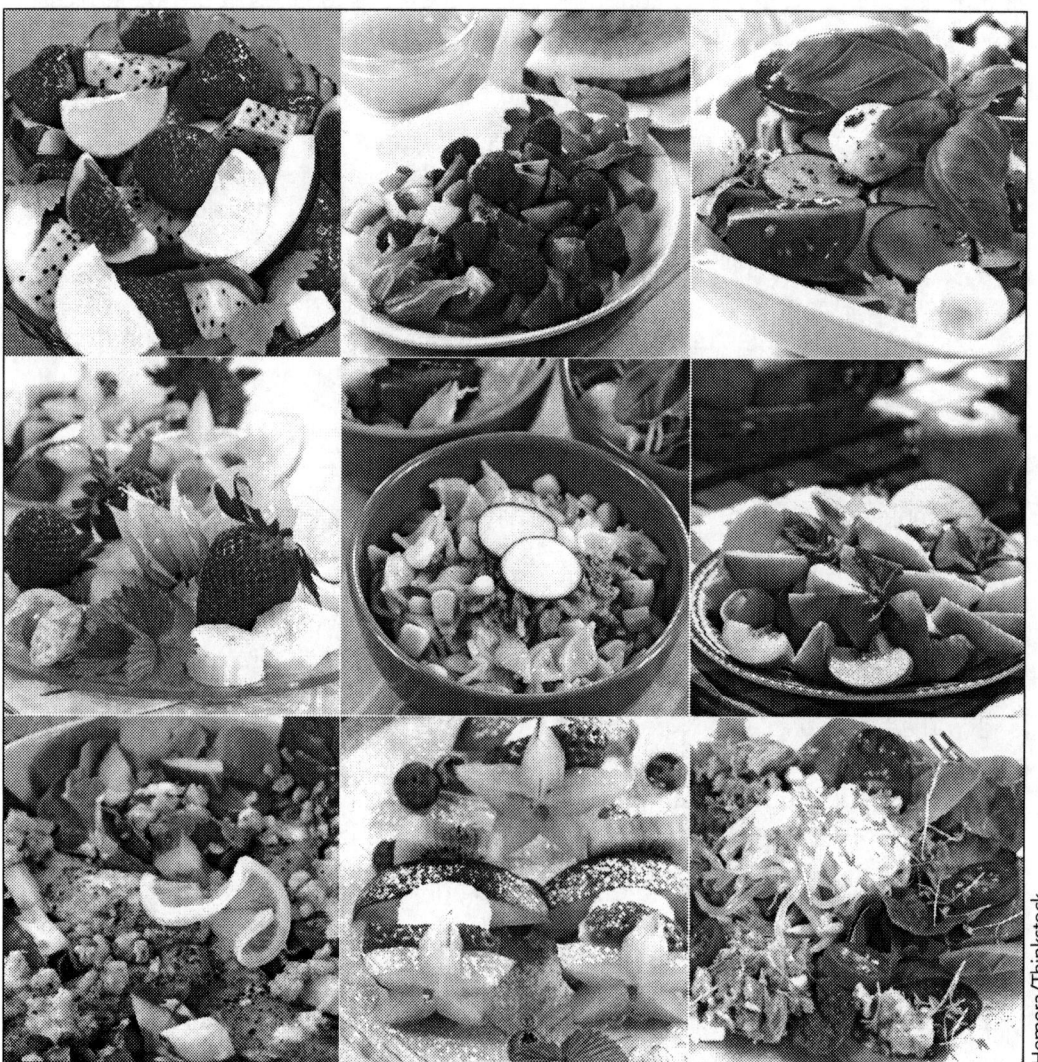

For overall good health, it is prudent to use whole foods to meet the optimal intakes of micronutrients (including antioxidants) and phytochemicals.

CHAPTER 7
HYDRATION—EVERYTHING YOU NEED TO KNOW ABOUT FLUIDS AND ELECTROLYTES

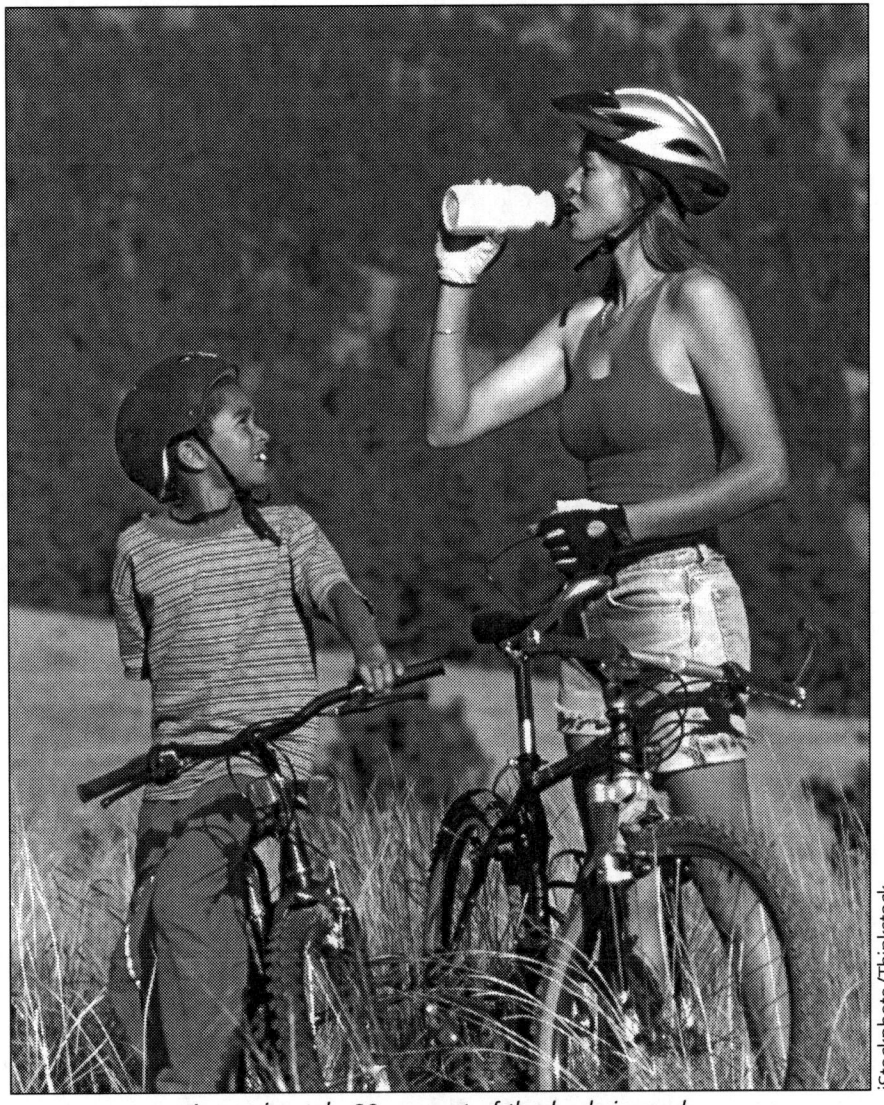

Approximately 60 percent of the body is made of water. Water is essential to survival.

Importance of Water

Approximately 60 percent of the body is made of water. Water is essential to survival and has the following functions:
- Transportation, as a component of blood and urine
- Removal of waste products
- Protection, serving as a lubricant, cleanser, and cushion
- Involvement in many metabolic reactions
- Temperature regulation (heat loss via sweat)

When a decrease in body water occurs, compensatory responses designed to conserve water take effect. One is decreased saliva production that causes dry mouth and increased thirst. Another is decreased blood volume that leads to decreased blood pressure that signals the brain to increase the thirst mechanism. The kidneys also play an important role by increasing water reabsorption in response to antidiuretic hormone.

Average body water loss is approximately 2.75 L per day. The apparent water losses occur in the form of sweat and urine at about 1 to 2 L per day, but an additional liter or so can be lost via evaporation in expired breath and from skin. The value is representative of an inactive person at room temperature. For an active person working in a warm environment, water losses can be much greater. The DRI for fluid intake in adults is 2.7 L per day for women and 3.7 L per day for men. These needs vary, depending on the level of physical activity and environmental conditions.

Physical Activity, Health, and Performance

Physical activity can induce increased sweat rates and, therefore, significantly higher water and electrolyte losses, with the magnitude of the losses being greater in a warm environment. Sweat rates vary greatly among individuals and with different types of physical activity. In general, women have lower sweat rates than men, but there may not be significant differences in electrolyte losses between the genders. Children may have lower sweat rates than adults, but the electrolyte losses may also be slightly lower or the same.

If water and electrolytes are not adequately replaced, dehydration will occur, which will result in impaired performance. Decreased body fluid levels at just over 2 percent of total body weight can lead to increased physiologic strain and perceived effort of the activity, especially in a warm environment. Though the data are not as abundant, dehydration that results in a 3 to 5 percent loss of body weight is unlikely to impair anaerobic or strength performance.

In addition to detriments in performance, dehydration can contribute to heat exhaustion and exertional heat stroke, and may increase the chance of developing, or the severity of, acute renal failure. Research data are less clear in supporting the relationship between dehydration and electrolyte loss and muscle cramps, but since fluids and electrolytes are necessary to maintain other physiological functions, it is prudent to ensure adequate intake of these two items.

Hydration Needs Before, During, and After Exercise

Beginning an exercise session or athletic event in a euhydrated (adequately hydrated) state is recommended for optimal performance. One of the simplest ways to determine the hydration level is by examining urine color. Urine that is clear or pale yellow is indicative of adequate hydration. If the urine darkens, dehydration is underway. Various urine color charts are available on the Internet and easily can be found using a search engine. To optimize water absorption and allow urine output to stabilize, it is best to begin consuming fluids several hours before physical activity. Beverages with electrolytes are valuable to stimulate thirst and help retain fluids in the body.

It is important to prevent, as much as possible, body-weight loss due to water loss during physical activity. To establish an accurate baseline body weight, a person must be in energy balance (weight stable) and be well hydrated. Body weight should be measured first thing in the morning, after urinating, and in the nude, for a minimum of three consecutive days. If daily weight is different by more than 1 percent, additional values should be taken, which is especially important for women, as they will experience body-water fluctuations with the menstrual cycle.

The hydration goal during physical activity is to maintain body weight within 2 percent of the baseline body weight. For example, a 125-pound female should drink enough to keep her body weight between 122.5 and 125 pounds after exercise. Because of variations in sweat rates and other factors—such as the duration of the activity, clothing and equipment, weather, and acclimatization to the environment—no one recommendation exists for all individuals and situations. A suggested starting point is 0.4 to 0.8 L of fluid per hour. In addition to consuming fluids and electrolytes during physical activity, the presence of carbohydrate in the beverage can help sustain endurance performance by sparing glycogen from being broken down in the body. The lower value for fluid intake (0.4 L) may be more appropriate for slower, smaller individuals, while the upper end (0.8 L) may be best for faster, larger people. Environment will also play a large factor. It is important to use pre- and post-exercise body weights during practice and training sessions to establish an individualized fluid replacement program. It is vital to plan ahead and practice beforehand since scales likely will not be available at all times.

Replacing fluid losses after exercise is a priority, but the first thing to consider is subsequent scheduled exercise sessions and athletic events. If an individual finishes a marathon and will not be engaging in further physical activity the rest of the day, adequate rehydration can be achieved by consuming beverages at meal times. On the other hand, situations may arise where more rapid rehydration is necessary. For example, when competing in a tournament, it is advisable to consume approximately 1.5 L of fluid for each kilogram lost and to continue to eat appropriate meals or snacks (preferably containing some sodium) throughout the day.

The Dangers of Hyponatremia

Hyponatremia is a general medical condition that involves having low serum sodium. Exercise-associated hyponatremia is specific to athletes and usually occurs with long-duration endurance events. Hyponatremia can be a severe medical condition that results in hospitalization or death. Hyponatremia generally occurs by overdrinking of hypotonic fluids (e.g., plain water) that is coupled with excessive sodium losses via sweat. The condition is more common in athletes with large sweat sodium losses who also have low body weights. It is beneficial to consume a sport drink before and during exercise because of the fluid, electrolytes, and carbohydrates supplied.

Beverage Choices

Water

Plain water can meet hydration needs when large amounts of sweat are not lost, as is the case with sedentary or light activities of short duration. The potential problem with plain water is taste—some people may not drink as much as is needed due to the lack of flavor. However, plain water is not appropriate for individuals who lose large amounts of sweat during activity due to the risk of developing hyponatremia. They need the additional electrolytes contained in sport drinks.

Traditional Sport Drinks

Most sport drinks are a 6 to 8 percent carbohydrate solution and generally contain approximately 14 to 15g of carbohydrate per cup. They also contain the electrolytes sodium, potassium, and chloride and should contain at least 70mg of sodium per cup. These beverages come in a variety of flavors, are inexpensive, readily accessible, and come in both powdered and liquid forms. Sport drinks are ideal for individuals exercising for longer periods of time (i.e., greater than 45 minutes) and are especially helpful in a warm environment.

Fitness Waters

Fitness waters are lightly flavored, but contain less carbohydrate (generally 3g per cup) and sodium than a traditional sport drink. People who sweat enough to need fluid replacement, but do not exercise intensely enough to warrant the carbohydrate content of the traditional sport drink, may benefit from using fitness waters. The added flavor in these products may encourage more fluid intake than plain water. Some current products have been fortified with calcium or have added caffeine. The caffeine content is modest and equivalent to diet colas (approximately 20mg of caffeine per cup). Many of these products are available in both liquid and powder form.

Specialized Sport Drinks

Some sport drinks may have a higher carbohydrate or sodium content than others. For example, individuals who have excessive sodium losses in their sweat may need a specialized product to optimally replenish these losses. Other specialty products contain only half of the carbohydrate content, and retain the same electrolyte concentration of traditional sport drinks. These products are ideal for times of intermittent high- and low-intensity exertion, as with sports that require engagement on the field and then some time off the field.

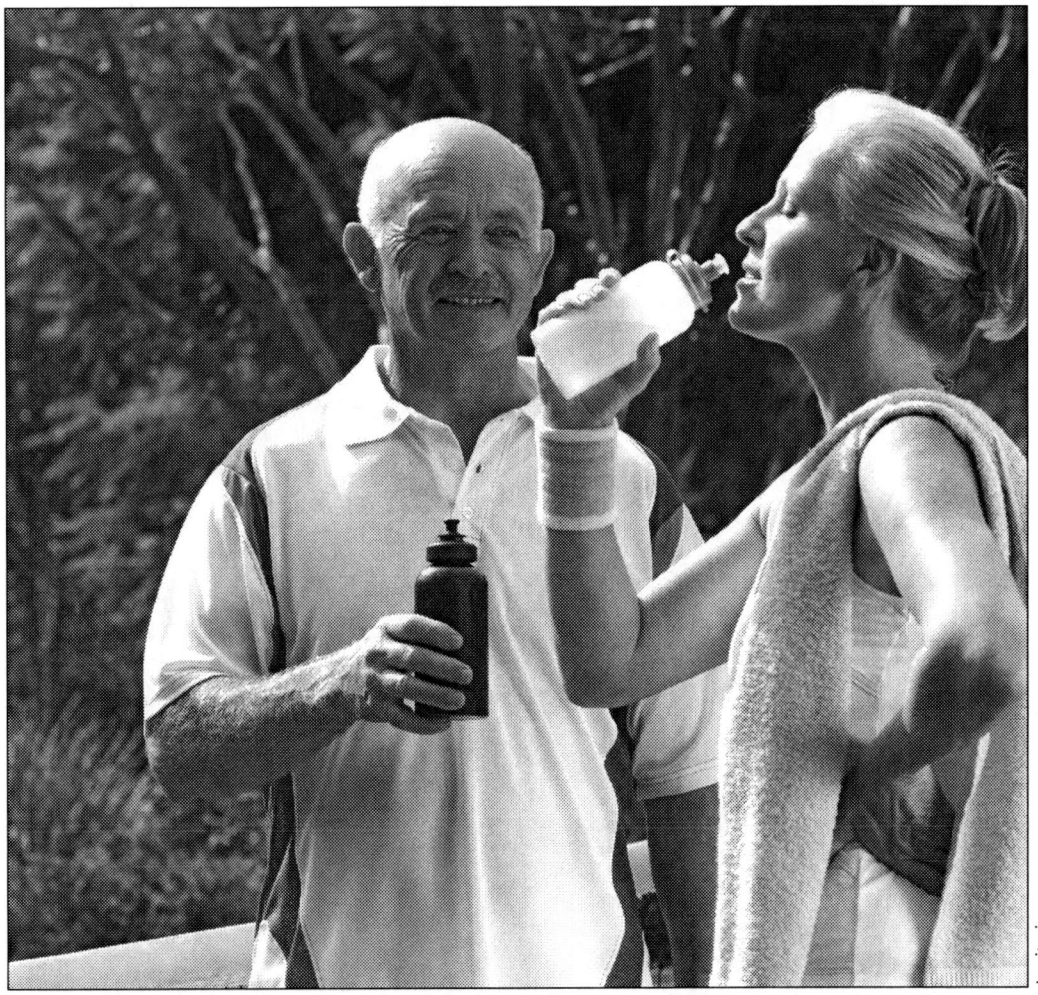

Some sport drinks may have a higher carbohydrate or sodium content than others.

Summary

Water has many functions, but a key one for athletes and physically active individuals is temperature regulation. Body weight losses of as little as 2 percent can impair endurance performance. It is important to prevent exercise-induced body-weight loss by consuming fluids before and after exercise. Sweat rates vary from person to person, and each individual must take responsibility for establishing a hydration schedule. Consuming fluids that contain electrolytes is important for the prevention of hyponatremia, and consuming fluids that contain carbohydrates is needed for the prevention of glycogen depletion and, therefore, enhanced endurance performance. Many beverages with added flavor are available that encourage fluid intake and replace the carbohydrate and electrolytes lost with physical exertion.

Section Three

Energy Balance and Weight Management

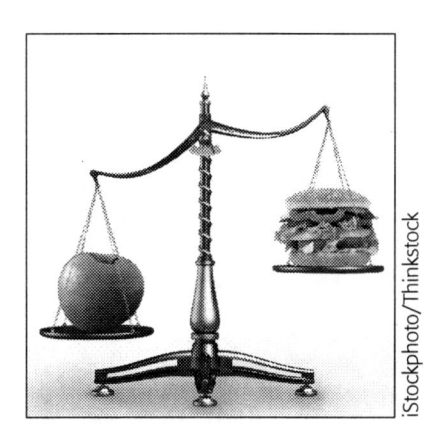

CHAPTER 8
ENERGY BALANCE

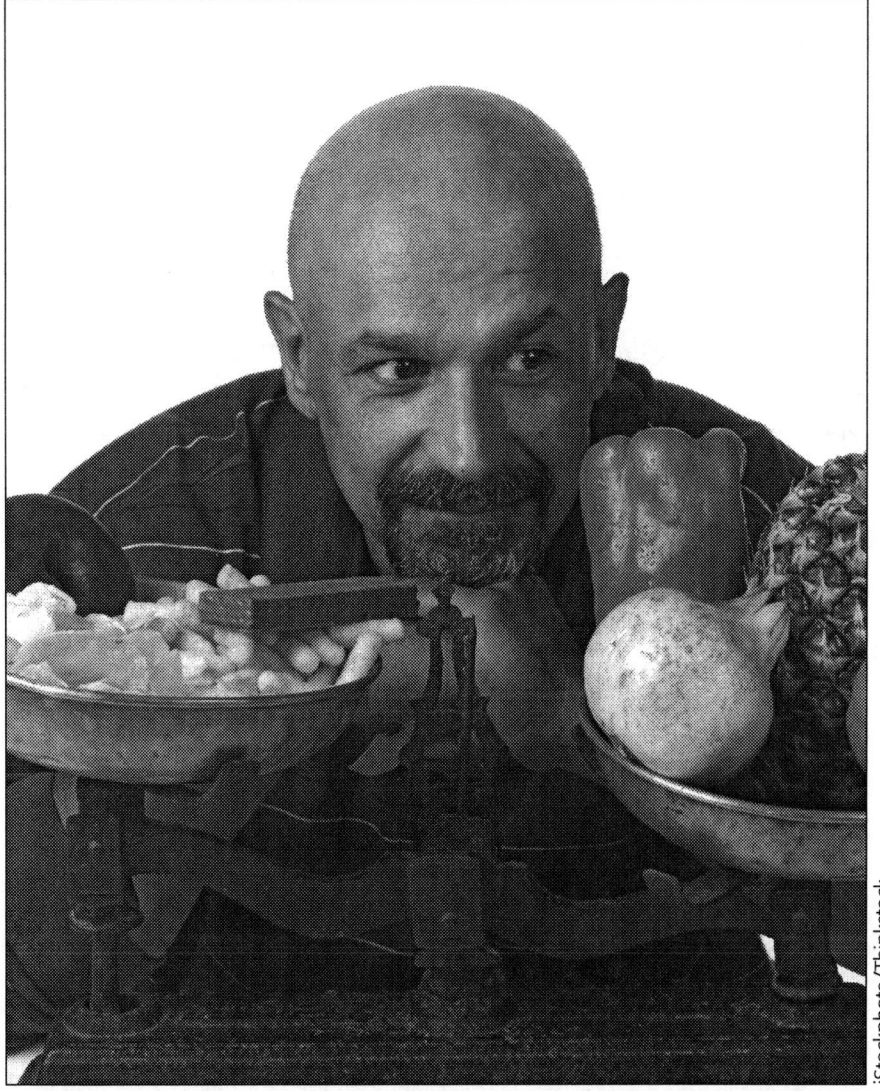

For a person to maintain body weight, there must be energy balance, or a situation in which energy consumed equals energy expended.

For a person to maintain body weight, there must be energy balance, or a situation in which energy consumed equals energy expended. If more energy is consumed than is used, weight will be gained; if more energy is expended than consumed, weight will be lost. It's that simple! However, numerous other factors contribute to and affect energy intake and expenditure. Several factors affect energy intake, such as ethnic and religious practices, family traditions, childhood experiences (e.g., foods received as rewards), emotional comfort received from food, access, convenience, availability, variety, education, occupation, income, nutrition beliefs, media or peer influences, and the taste of food. Some factors may not be easily controllable—such as physical disability, injury or other form of activity restriction, and physical environment (e.g., living in an unsafe neighborhood)—while other factors, such as making time for exercise, may be. Although it is relatively easy to describe the concept of energy balance, it is much more difficult to implement it in practice.

Components of Energy Expenditure

Total daily energy expenditure (TDEE) can be broken down into the following three components:

- Resting metabolic rate (RMR), also known as resting energy expenditure (REE)
- Thermic effect of food (TEF), also known as dietary induced thermogenesis (DIT)
- Energy expenditure due to physical activity (EEPA)

Resting Metabolic Rate

RMR, the largest component of the TDEE, represents 60 to 75 percent of daily expenditure and is the amount of energy the body expends on maintenance activities while at rest, such as growth and maintenance of tissues, organ function, breathing, circulation, and other bodily activities that keep people alive. Many years of scientific research indicate that a key factor correlated with RMR is lean body mass (LBM), which is made up of muscle, bone, and water. The common saying that "muscle burns more calories than fat" is actually true. Maintaining skeletal muscle requires approximately 13 kcal/kg per day, while adipose tissue requires only 4.5 kcal/kg per day. One effective way to increase RMR is to build skeletal muscle through resistance training. While organs also significantly contribute to RMR, their size or activity cannot be healthily influenced through training or lifestyle modifications and, therefore, will not be discussed further.

Thermic Effect of Food

TEF is the energy expended to digest and metabolize food. TEF is the smallest component of TDEE, representing only 5 to 10 percent of the total. Because many factors affect this component, TEF needs to be examined carefully. For example, the TEF is a little higher when digesting and metabolizing proteins and carbohydrates as compared to fats. However, this does not mean that unlimited quantities of protein or carbohydrate can be consumed without weight gain. Similarly, TEF is higher for a larger meal as compared with a small snack, but energy expenditure is not significant enough to warrant the frequent consumption of large meals.

Some fad diet books claim that the timing and/or combinations of nutrient consumption will maximize TEF. While the scientific data may support this conclusion to an extent, the clinical significance of this theory makes it not entirely worthwhile to attempt to control. Eating these combinations may lead to an increased TEF of only 25 calories per day. It is likely easier to take an extra flight or two of stairs or consume one less piece of hard candy to account for those 25 calories. In addition, measuring TEF is impractical and it is difficult to detect if it is working. Emphasis needs to be placed on the larger picture: decreasing total energy intake and increasing energy expenditure via physical activity.

Energy Expenditure Due to Physical Activity

EEPA represents all voluntary physical activity, including structured exercise, informal activities (e.g., gardening, running errands, housework), and even fidgeting. EEPA is the most variable of the three components of energy expenditure, typically representing 15 to 30 percent of the TDEE in most individuals. EEPA can also fall outside of this range. For example, EEPA in a very sedentary person may fall below 15 percent, while in an elite endurance athlete in training it may be greater than 30 percent. Of the three components of TDEE, EEPA is the one that is most controllable (unless a limiting physical disability is present). EPPA is the component where a fitness professional can be most influential with helping you achieve weight-management goals.

Measuring Energy Intake and Expenditure

The overarching goal of weight management is balance energy intake with energy expenditure. On the energy intake side of the balance equation, the dietician's role is to help clients understand the energy content of the foods consumed and how to best determine this information. On the energy expenditure side, it is the fitness professional's role to determine the mode, frequency, intensity, and duration of physical activity to best meet your weight-management goals.

The energy content of food is measured by a laboratory technique called bomb calorimetry. A sample of dried food is burned, and the amount of heat given off is measured in units called kilocalories (kcal). The kilocalories are in the form of gross energy, which does not take digestibility into consideration. However, the energy values that appear on a food label or in a nutrient database do take digestibility factors into account, and the information can be comfortably used by consumers. For example, foods high in fiber are not fully digested in a human body, but are completely combusted in a bomb calorimeter. Therefore, the amount of kilocalories shown on a food label or listed in the USDA nutrient database is invariably less than those measured in a bomb calorimeter.

Similar to how heat emission from food burned in a bomb calorimeter is used to determine its energy content, heat production during physical activity is used to estimate energy expenditure in a room calorimeter. This direct measure of energy expenditure is accurate; however, due to its high cost and relative scarcity, it is rarely used in practice. An alternative method to direct calorimetry involves the collection of inspired and expired air and subsequent analysis of oxygen consumption and carbon dioxide production during rest or physical activity. This method is used widely in both research and clinical practice.

Any wellness professional who agrees to help you achieve your weight-management goals must be able to program a suitable level of exercise to balance your energy-intake level. A personal trainer is *not* qualified to provide nutritional advice unless he has had significant additional training and certification in this area.

While performing a complete nutrition assessment is not usually within the scope of practice for a fitness professional, it is within the scope of a dietician.

The estimates are a good starting point to determine how much to eat in order to meet goals (i.e., weight loss or maintenance) or how many calories are burned during an exercise session. If weight gain or weight loss is occurring, then you are not in energy balance, even if the equations indicate otherwise. The next step would be to adjust the exercise program or energy needs estimate accordingly. In addition to the fitness professional's guidance, you can use the MyPlate website to track energy balance for up to one year.

Summary

If your weight is stable, then you are in energy balance. The three components of total daily energy expenditure are resting metabolic rate, thermic effect of food, and energy expenditure due to physical activity. Resting metabolic rate is the largest component of total expenditure, but physical activity is the most variable. Both energy content of food and energy expenditure can be estimated using various techniques.

CHAPTER 9
WEIGHT-LOSS PRINCIPLES

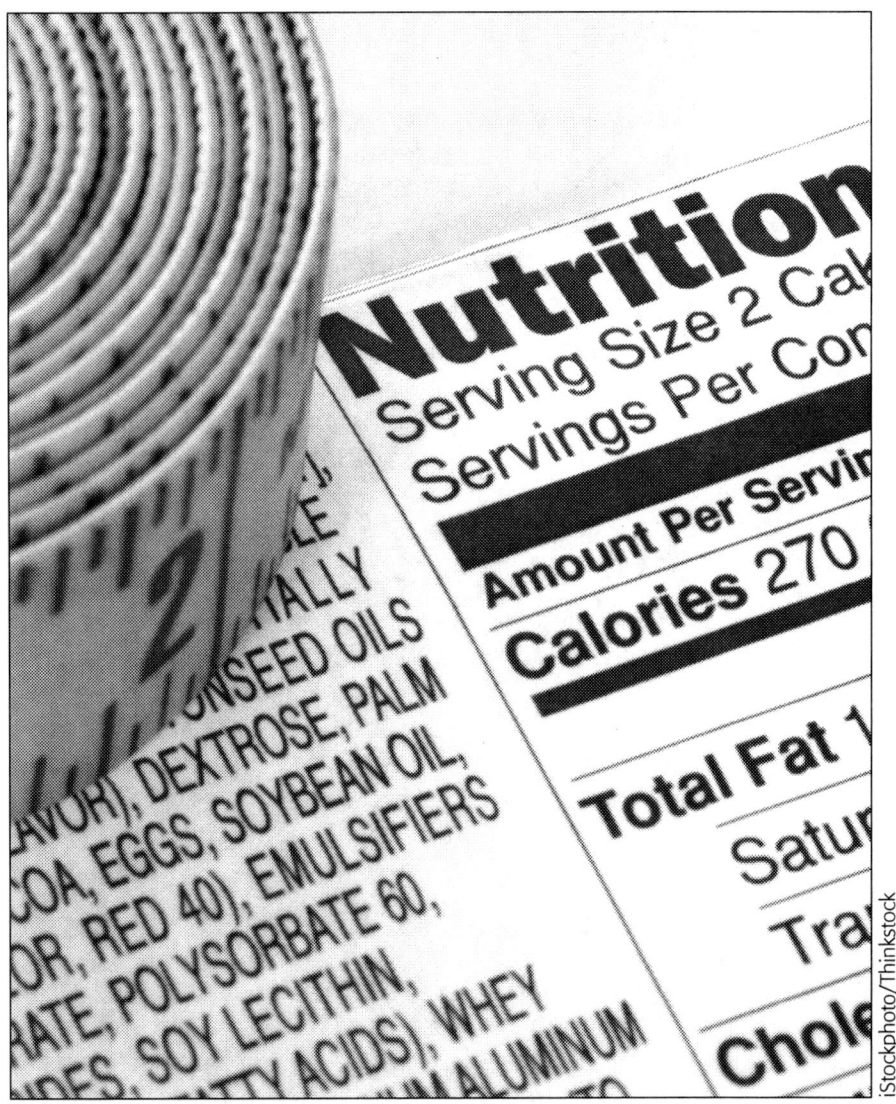

Sound weight-loss plans are those that control energy intake and promote regular physical activity, while instilling lifelong changes in habits.

The health consequences of being overweight or obese are available from many sources. According to the Centers for Disease Control, 65 percent of American adults are overweight or obese, with an average weight gain of 1.75 pounds (0.8 kg) each year. Overweight or obesity is associated with an increased risk for many chronic diseases, including the following:

- Type 2 diabetes
- Hypertension
- Dyslipidemia and cardiovascular disease
- Gallbladder disease
- Osteoarthritis
- Some cancers
- Sleep apnea

One way of defining overweight and obesity in an individual is the use of the body mass index (BMI). While BMI has limitations when used in some individuals, it is a reasonable tool to use when categorizing overweight and obesity in populations; a BMI of 25 to 29.9 is considered overweight, while a BMI of 30 or greater is indicative of obesity.

Both environmental and genetic factors contribute to obesity. While research is in the early stages, it appears that several physiological factors also play a role. For example, adipose tissue is not only a stagnant place to store fat. It appears to secrete hormones, such as leptin, which may play a role in satiety. Another hormone secreted by the stomach, ghrelin, may contribute to obesity by increasing appetite. Genetics may play a role as well. The offspring of normal-weight parents have a 10 percent chance of becoming obese. If one or both parents are obese, this chance is increased to 40 percent or 80 percent, respectively.

While genetics and physiology contribute to body-weight regulation, the population-wide weight gain seen in the United States is also likely due to cultural influences that encourage a chronic energy imbalance due to excess food intake and/or decreased physical activity. A strong inverse relationship exists between obesity and levels of physical activity and fitness levels; less active and unfit individuals have a greater risk for becoming obese. Similarly, people who engage in more physical activity and are fit tend to gain less weight over time.

Principles of Weight Management

As previously indicated, energy balance is critical for weight management. While being out of balance for a short time will not lead to significant weight changes, chronic energy imbalance will lead to weight loss or gain. Though the statement that 3,500 calories equals one pound of fat is not 100 percent metabolically accurate, it is close and useful for our purposes. To lose a pound of fat in one week, a person must be in an energy deficit of 500 calories per day (3,500 calories/seven days). The deficit can be achieved through reduced energy intake, increased energy expenditure, or, ideally, both. Similarly, a person wanting to gain weight (muscle mass) needs to consume an additional 400 to 500 calories per day and participate in an appropriate strength-training regimen. While a simple concept in theory, implementing it may not be easy.

Sound weight-loss plans are those that control energy intake and promote regular physical activity, while instilling lifelong changes in habits. Individuals seeking to lose weight may not recognize that the weight gain possibly took years, and may expect weight loss to be quick and easy. This perspective is not surprising considering all of the media claims about how easy weight loss can be with a particular diet or pill. Sometimes, it can be challenging to convince yourself that lifelong habit changes are crucial for weight loss and maintenance. A sound weight-loss plan generally has the following characteristics:

- Promotes a slow and steady weight loss (e.g., one pound per week)
- A weight loss of approximately 10 percent of body weight is followed by a three- to six-month period of weight maintenance
- Encourages common foods
- Allows the individual to participate in social events and eat at restaurants
- Allows flexibility for individual food preferences
- Restricts energy while other nutrient needs are met
- Promotes lifelong changes in habits
- Includes social support
- Does not eliminate certain foods or whole food groups
- Is science-based
- Encourages regular physical activity

As we have mentioned throughout the book, there are no bad foods and there is no one perfect strategy for each and every person. However, there are some precautions that everyone should consider when they hear of the perfect diet plan that promotes the use of weight loss supplements, requires the purchase of special foods, or makes unrealistic claims.

Fad Diets

When people want to lose weight, one of the first things they turn to is a popular diet, and, with many diet books on the shelves and diet plans on the Internet, it can be overwhelming. In addition, many diet books and plans promise to be the last diet a person will ever need and that the unwanted pounds will melt away. If losing weight was as easy as these diets claim, the obesity epidemic in this county would be a nonissue. The following is a summary of some of the more popular diets that are promoted by personalities and the print media or somehow go viral on the Internet.

Carbohydrate-Restricted Diets

Carbohydrate-restricted diets vary in the amount of the daily carbohydrate "allowed," but the amount often ranges from 20 to 90 grams per day. These diets usually allow unlimited protein and fat. The common claims in these diets are that consuming carbohydrates leads to weight gain and that insulin is an undesirable anabolic hormone that promotes fat storage. Is it a true statement that eating carbohydrates will make people fat? It is only partially true. Carbohydrates will lead to weight gain if more are consumed than the body burns for fuel or stores as glycogen, but making a blanket statement that consuming carbohydrates leads to a gain in body fat is inappropriate. Consider elite runners. They are not fat, but they do eat lots of carbohydrate. However, elite runners burn what is consumed. If more carbohydrate is consumed than is being used, the anabolic hormone insulin will promote fat storage. The books and diets that promote carbohydrate restriction fail to mention that insulin also plays a role in skeletal muscle protein synthesis.

Do these diets work? If you look at simply pounds lost, then the answer is a resounding "yes" in the first 7 to 10 days. The problem is that much of the weight reduction is due to loss of body water, not body fat. With restricted carbohydrate intake, glycogen becomes depleted, and body water is lost. For every gram of glycogen stored in the body, almost 3 grams of water is stored with it. The glycogen stores are used in the initial days of the diet, which will result in water loss. The outcomes of a few short-term studies have reported more weight loss with low-carbohydrate diets. However, studies that are longer (6 to 12 months) show no benefit of a low-carbohydrate diet over other types of diets. According to these studies, the key factors for weight loss were energy restriction and exercise. A few more recent studies have examined the role of protein, independent of carbohydrate intake, on weight loss. Some preliminary data suggest that higher protein intakes (still within the DRI) may be associated with slight increases in energy expenditure, which may result in greater satiation. More data are needed before absolute conclusions can be made.

Are there any adverse health effects to consuming a low-carbohydrate diet? The answer to this question is not quite clear. In the short-term, it is unlikely, but, due to the lack of well-controlled, long-term research studies, less is known about chronic reduced consumption. When carbohydrate intake is restricted to the point that glycogen stores are depleted, the body will try to use fat for fuel. Carbohydrate is needed for the complete breakdown of a fatty acid molecule. When carbohydrate is not available, the fatty acid molecules will partially break down, and then turn to an alternate, available pathway. The result is the formation of ketone bodies. While the brain and nervous tissue function better with carbohydrate as a fuel source, ketones can be used as a backup fuel. Because ketones are acids, excessive production of ketones is considered unhealthy and could lead to ketoacidosis, a dangerous metabolic condition that can result in coma or death. Fortunately, the ketone levels from dietary carbohydrate restriction usually do not reach the dangerous levels that are seen in a person with diabetes. People trying to adhere to the limits in the carbohydrate-restricted diets sometimes may consume additional carbohydrates, keeping the ketone levels reasonable. Ketones also help suppress appetite, which may lead to some people still choosing this method of dieting.

While ketones can be used to an extent as a fuel source, the brain and nervous tissue still need some glucose. As previously noted, glucose cannot be synthesized from fatty acids (only a small amount from the glycerol backbone). However, glucose can be synthesized from glucogenic amino acids. It is unclear how carbohydrate-restricted diets affect body composition. Is the protein consumed in the diet being used to make glucose instead of other items? Is skeletal muscle being catabolized to make glucose for the brain in the absence of carbohydrate? More research studies are needed before these questions can be accurately answered.

Some health consequences may occur from following the diet, specifically related to the development of chronic disease. If the diet is high in healthy fats (poly- and monounsaturated), then hyperlipidemia may not be an issue. If, however, a large amount of saturated or trans fats are consumed, then dyslipidemia may be a side effect. While studies have shown these diets do not have a negative effect on blood lipids, limitations exist. The studies were short-term in length, and, therefore, the effects of adhering to this type of diet long-term are unknown. Furthermore, the factor of weight loss itself must be considered. If a person loses weight, no matter what method is used, serum cholesterol generally will be lowered. It is less clear whether or not this drop in serum cholesterol will be maintained, and more importantly, whether it translates to a reduced risk of developing cardiovascular disease. More research studies are needed in this area, and other factors that may influence the serum lipid profile, such as heredity, dietary intake, and physical-activity patterns, need to be examined. Another factor to consider is that these diets can fail to provide adequate amounts of some key nutrients for health, including calcium, magnesium, potassium, antioxidants, and phytochemicals. No concrete answers are available to define the relationship between diet and cancer. However, some data exist that support that populations who consume diets high in animal products and low in plant foods have an increased risk for developing some cancers. The Dietary Approaches to Stop Hypertension (DASH, www.dashdiet.org) trials showed that diets moderate in sodium, and rich in fruits and vegetables, and that include low-fat dairy and lean protein were effective in improving blood pressure. The low-carbohydrate diets lack many of these nutrients. Diets that are more carbohydrate controlled (rather than carbohydrate restricted) generally promote intake of quality carbohydrates, lean protein sources, and healthy fats. However, some plans still have restrictions of certain foods or food groups without any scientific rationale.

Some limitations exist with the currently available studies. First, one macronutrient level cannot be manipulated without affecting another one (if one is increased, another is decreased). In this case, it is difficult to attribute any weight changes to one of the nutrients. Second, leaner individuals lose more lean body mass per unit of body weight than those who have more body fat. Furthermore, men may lose more lean body mass per unit of body weight than women. It is important for research studies to have well-matched subjects if weight loss or body composition is a study outcome.

Until strong research data support a different recommendation for weight loss, it is wise to consume carbohydrate, fat, and protein ratios consistent with the following current DRIs for macronutrients: 45 to 65 percent carbohydrate, 10 to 35 percent protein, and 20 to 35 percent fat. Adequate protein intake (within the DRI range) coupled with resistance training may help maintain lean body mass during periods of weight loss. The wide ranges allow for individual responses to macronutrient patterns and encourage individual meal-planning choices.

Food Combining

Some diet plans emphasize that eating specific foods in the proper combination will result in weight loss. For example, many plans promote not consuming carbohydrates, fats, or proteins at the same time because the digestive enzymes responsible for these nutrients will cancel each other out and the digestive process will be altered. If not digested in the small intestine, then carbohydrates, fats, and proteins go to the large intestine and, ultimately, out of the body. Any macronutrient not absorbed in the small intestine will eventually be excreted in the feces. From a weight-loss standpoint, it would be great to be able to eat carbohydrates, proteins, and fats at the same time and have the calories canceled out. Some of these diets take it further and suggest that beverage consumption, specifically water, with meals dilutes the digestive enzymes and renders them ineffective. If this were true, a large meal of pizza and soda could be consumed, and the calories would filter through the body without affecting it. In fact, water is already present in the digestive tract to aid in the digestive process and is then reabsorbed into the body. If it were possible, this diet method would certainly be a very unhealthy mode of weight loss, but in some sense a dream to the dieter. Notwithstanding the fact that there are no research data to support this concept, it physiologically does not make sense.

Weight Loss vs. Weight Maintenance

Most fad diets will result in weight loss because they are inherently low in calories. In addition, many individuals trying to lose weight can tolerate food restrictions for short periods of time. While it is a proven fact that obesity is associated with the risk of developing many chronic diseases and that weight loss can improve health, some individuals may not consider the importance of weight maintenance. Many people can lose weight for a time, but what percentage of those who do are able to keep the weight off? Given the current obesity epidemic, it seems that few individuals succeed at weight-loss maintenance.

Some of the most compelling data available at this time come from the National Weight Control Registry (NWCR, www.nwcr.ws). The NWCR, created in 1994, is the largest research investigation of successful weight loss maintenance. The NWCR has data on more than 5,000 individuals who have lost significant amounts of weight and maintained that weight loss for extended periods of time. The overall conclusion thus far is that the successful participants in the study have two common courses of action: dietary and physical-activity modification. Dietary modification includes changes like eating breakfast daily and using portion control, while the physical-activity patterns include exercising approximately one hour per day and watching television less than 10 hours per week. Regular body-weight measurements also seem to be a motivating factor.

Although little data are available to support fad diets, some strong evidence exists to support lifestyle changes, such as portion control and regular physical activity.

Limitations With Fad Diets

No significant scientific research exists to support a specific fad diet plan. In fad diets, the ease of weight loss is promised, often without exercise, and foods or food groups are forbidden or restricted. The diets may be inadequate for health and balanced nutrition. They are also generally hard to plan for, since changes in habits are required overnight and participants are encouraged to follow the rules rather than develop habits that can be sustained long term.

Any diet book or plan that promotes easy weight loss without exercise should be viewed with caution. Fortunately, many good books and plans are available that teach sensible eating strategies with an emphasis on macronutrient balance and portion control. The DRIs and MyPlate are excellent resources for healthy individuals to use for assessing their personal energy balance and developing a portion-controlled meal plan on their own. Someone with a disease or other medical condition (e.g., diabetes, cardiovascular disease, or hypertension) who is seeking weight-loss advice should consult a registered dietitian for individualized meal planning.

Weight Loss and Body Composition

From the available literature on diets, it appears that the macronutrient distribution is not as important as total energy intake when attempting to lose weight. In addition to total weight loss, it is important to consider the composition of the weight lost. A negative energy balance results in weight loss from a reduction in both fat mass and lean body mass, with the losses of lean body mass being significant with more severe energy restriction.

Some individuals wanting to lose weight may have the goal of reducing body fat while simultaneously gaining lean body mass, specifically muscle mass. It would be difficult to achieve this goal because dieting puts the body in a state of catabolism, but to facilitate muscle mass gain, the body needs to be in a state of anabolism. It is prudent to work toward an appropriate weight loss (1 to 2 pounds per week) through modest energy restriction and physical activity. An example of this would be to create a 500 kcal/day energy deficit by reducing energy intake and increasing energy expenditure.

Some individuals may want to lose weight very quickly and turn to low-calorie meal plans to accomplish this goal. In this case, the proportion of lean body mass loss may be greater than body-fat loss. A higher percent body fat may result even though body weight was lost. This relative increase in fat with the concomitant reduction in lean body mass may be discouraging to those individuals trying to lose weight.

As mentioned previously, weight loss is easier to accomplish than weight maintenance. The following are general strategies for successful weight loss and weight maintenance:

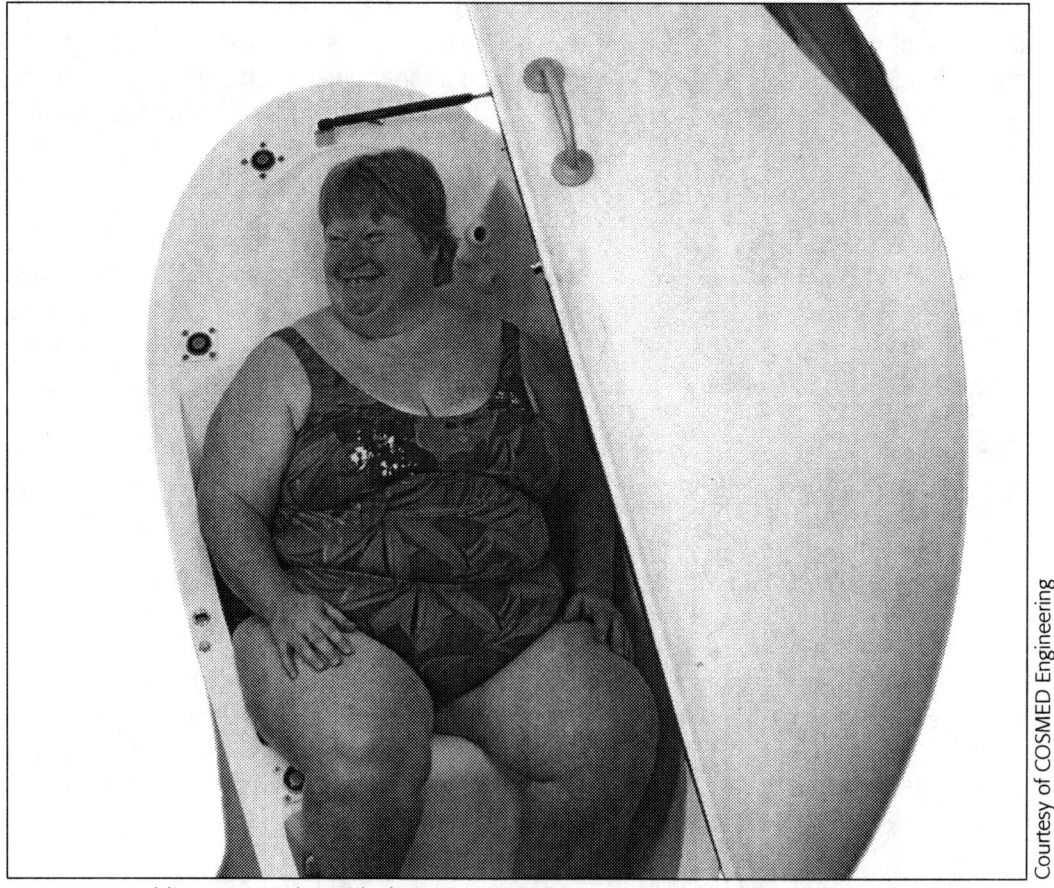

In addition to total weight loss, it is important to consider the composition of the weight lost. One method for assessing body composition is the BOD POD.

- *Initial weight loss goals should be approximately 10 percent of body weight.* This loss should be achieved through a modest energy deficit (e.g., 500 kcal/day) created by calorie control and increased physical activity.
- *Once 10 percent of the body weight is lost, ideally the person should work to maintain that weight loss for approximately three months.* Once the three months are finished, the person can reevaluate his body weight and set a new goal of 10 percent weight loss. Individuals seeking to lose weight may want to lose as much weight as possible in the shortest amount of time. By losing weight in stages, they are more likely to develop permanent lifestyle habits that translate into long-term body-weight maintenance.
- *Regular physical activity may not result in a simultaneous decrease in body fat and increase in lean body mass.* However, an appropriate exercise program consisting of aerobic exercise and strength training can increase the likelihood of maintaining lean body mass during the energy deficit period.

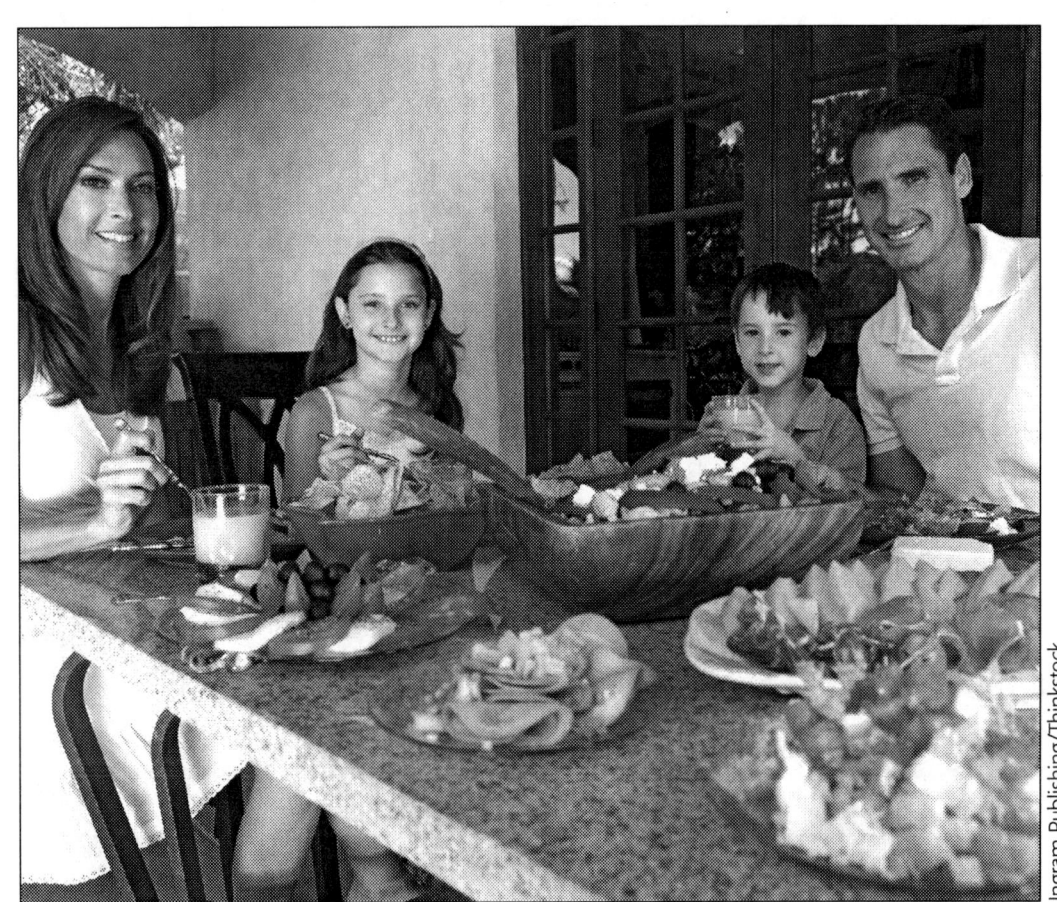

All factors considered, weight loss is easier to accomplish than weight maintenance.

Weight Cycling

Weight cycling occurs when people experience repeating periods of weight loss and weight gain. Usually, people who are motivated by the diet fad of the month are initially intrigued by the novelty, experience no long-term habit changes, and, ultimately, go back to their old habits. When people lose weight, they lose not only fat, but also lean body mass, especially if exercise is not part of the plan. When they gain the weight back, it is primarily in the form of fat, assuming that exercise is still not part of the lifestyle. This chronic loss of lean body mass and gain of body fat results in an altered body composition such that after years of weight cycling, body weight may be the same, but the percent body fat is higher. This alteration in body composition will likely make it even harder to lose or maintain weight because resting metabolism may also be lowered. It is better to lose a few pounds and maintain it for a long period than to chronically lose and gain larger quantities of body mass.

Weight-Loss Supplements

Similar to the promises of diet books, many claims are made by supplement manufacturers regarding easy weight loss—no counting calories, and, often, no required exercise.

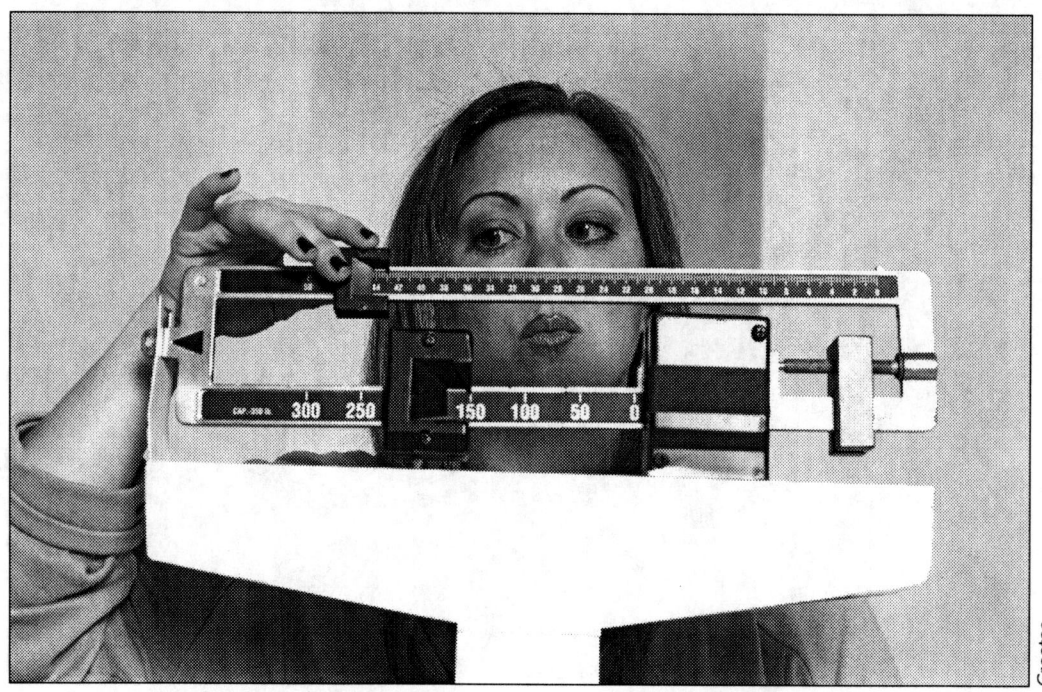

When people lose weight, they lose not only fat, but also lean body mass, especially if exercise is not part of the plan.

Carnitine

Carnitine is a compound that aids the transport of fatty acids across the mitochondrial membrane for oxidation (breakdown). The theory is that ingesting the compound results in increased fatty acid oxidation, and hence fat loss. The body naturally makes carnitine, and research data do not support its effectiveness in increasing fat loss.

Chromium Picolinate

Chromium is a trace mineral required for insulin action and is often promoted for weight loss. Well-designed studies using up to 1,000 μg/day of the mineral do not show a significant effect on weight loss. A UL has not yet been determined for chromium, but some studies reported potentially serious side effects and, therefore, caution should be used when consuming more than 200 μg per day. While this supplement appears ineffective for weight loss, limited data suggest a potential for blood glucose improvements in people with type 2 diabetes. The key here is that chromium may be beneficial only in conjunction with weight management, carbohydrate control, and physical activity, not as a substitute for these lifestyle modifications.

Pyruvate

Pyruvate is the end product of glycolysis and is often promoted for weight loss. Research is limited, but a few studies show a small effect on weight loss when large doses of pyruvate are ingested, usually in combination with large doses of the compound dihydroxyacetone (DHA). Common doses of pyruvate generally rage from 1 to 3g/day, whereas the research studies used up to 30g/day with up to 75g of DHA. Taking these doses would be quite expensive. Data are insufficient to report on the safety of this supplement.

Chitosan

Proponents for chitosan claim that it binds to dietary fat in the intestine and, thus, prevent fats absorption. Only a few published studies that used this product reported small differences in weight loss. Since the product is supposed to bind to fat in the digestive tract and eliminate it, it would follow that an increase in fecal fat would occur. Interestingly, one study examined fecal fat with use of chitosan and found it to be clinically insignificant in men and nonexistent in women. Some gastrointestinal side effects have been reported, such as flatulence, nausea, vomiting, and diarrhea.

Conjugated Linoleic Acid

The compound conjugated linoleic acid (CLA) has several isomers, and it is believed that the two with the most biological activity are cis-9, trans-11 and trans-10, cis-12. Quite a few published animal studies report positive effects of CLA supplementation on fat loss and reduced energy consumption. It does seem that different species respond best to different isomers. However, some side effects have been seen in the animal studies such as insulin resistance and increased liver and spleen weight. The data in humans are not as promising, and not enough data exist to support its use for fat loss. More data are needed on appropriate isomers and doses in humans.

Hydroxycitric Acid

Manufacturers of the supplement hydoxycitric acid (HCA) claim it is a stimulant and inhibits lipogenesis. A few animal studies have shown decreased food intake and weight regain after weight loss. The few studies in humans have mixed results; some studies showed small effects on weight loss while others showed none. More data are needed before conclusions can be made about the safety and efficacy of this product.

Tea

The media promotion of green tea for weight loss has increased. It is believed that the active compounds in some teas—the powerful antioxidant epigallocatechin gallate (EGCG) and caffeine—may act to promote weight loss. Studies have been completed mostly with green and oolong teas, and some suggest small increases in fat oxidation, energy expenditure, and weight loss with consumption. These positive data are still sparse and should be interpreted with caution. It is important to understand that for people who are very sensitive to caffeine, consuming excessive amounts of tea can result in side effects. In addition, caffeine in high doses may be a banned substance for competitive athletes by their governing organization.

Ma Huang/Ephedra/Ephedrine

Ma huang (also known as ephedra or ephedrine) was banned for sale in the United States by the Federal Drug Administration (FDA) in April 2004. Rigorous reviews of research studies do report modest increases in short-term weight loss with this product. However, the potential psychiatric, autonomic, and cardiac side effects were significant. It is important to emphasize that the possible small increases in weight loss are not worth the potential side effects of using the product, which may still be available for purchase in other countries.

Citrus Aurantium

Now that ephedra/ephedrine products have been banned, citrus aurantium (CA) is a common ingredient in weight-loss products that claim to be "ephedra-free" or "ephedrine-free." It is also known as bitter orange or sour orange. The plant extract contains m-synephrine and phenylephrine, and it is believed that these are the active, stimulatory ingredients that aid in weight loss. The research on this compound is very scarce, and the few studies that have been done combined CA with ephedra/ephedrine, St. John's Wort, and/or caffeine, with one of these studies reporting greater weight loss with the product. The following question remains: Is it the CA itself or the CA acting with other compounds that results in the small increases in weight loss? Two studies did report a possible association between CA and cardiovascular side effects. More data are needed on this product before its efficacy or safety can be discussed with confidence.

Calcium and Weight Loss

Media promotion of dairy foods for weight loss has increased and, therefore, understanding this relationship is important. One theory behind calcium and weight loss is as follows: Low calcium intake is associated with activation of Vitamin D (1, 25-dihydroxyvitamin D), which in turn increases calcium deposition into the adipose tissue and pancreatic cells. When calcium concentrations increase in these cells, it promotes fatty acid synthesis and inhibits breakdown. Consuming adequate calcium would prevent these cellular changes and have the opposite effect on lipid metabolism. There is not enough scientific research to suggest this mechanism is fact. It's an interesting theory being investigated in many laboratories around the world—but for now it's just a theory.

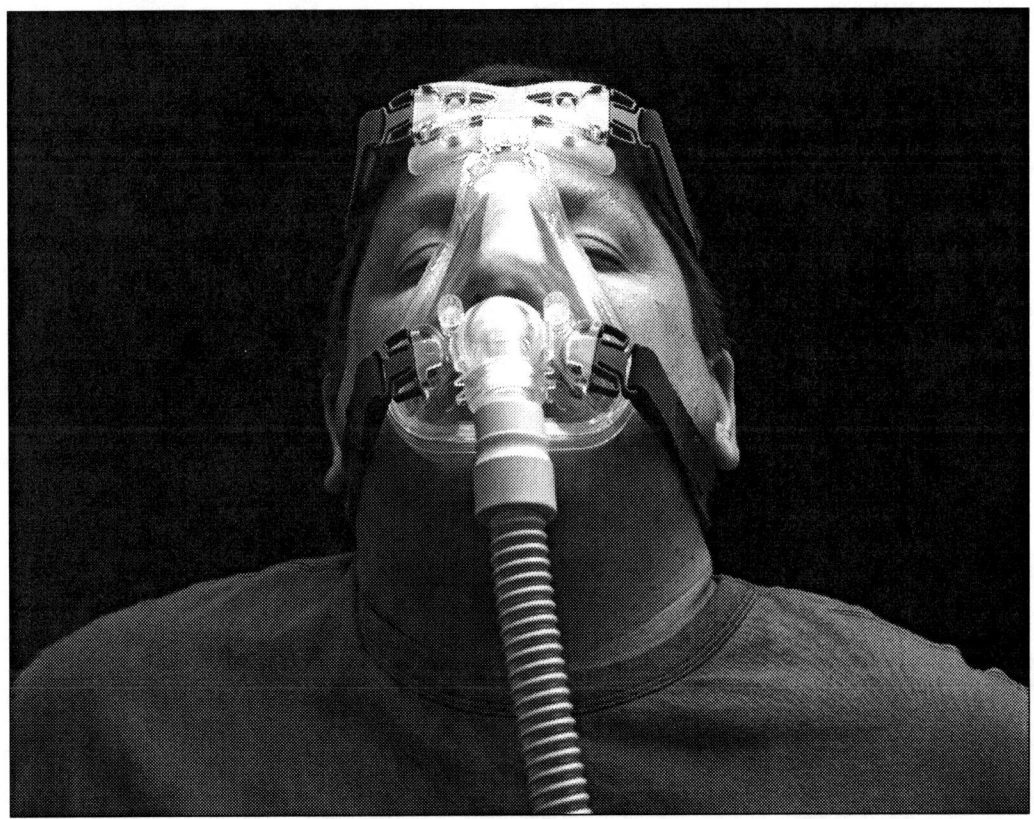

Overweight and obesity are conditions associated with an increased risk of many chronic diseases and medical complications.

Several epidemiological studies have examined the relationship between calcium intake and body weight and/or body fat and reported a negative association between the two variables. In the studies, groups of people who had lower calcium intakes have higher body weights than groups who consumed adequate or higher calcium. In addition to the population studies, two clinical trials have been published examining calcium intake and weight loss. One study concluded that three dairy servings a day resulted in more total and abdominal fat loss than calcium in the supplemental form or little daily intake of dairy products. All three groups were in a 500 kcal/day energy-restricted state. Another study reported that those eating three servings of yogurt per day, compared to a control group, experienced significantly more total fat loss and trunk fat loss.

Summary

Overweight and obesity are conditions associated with an increased risk of many chronic diseases and medical complications. Both genetic and environmental factors are related to body weight and body fat. While genetic factors cannot be controlled, environmental factors can be. Two of the key environmental factors that influence body weight are food intake and physical activity.

Sound weight-management plans include controlling energy intake and regular physical activity in such a way to induce lifelong changes in habits. Hundreds of fad diets and plans are available and yet, oftentimes, very little scientific evidence exists to support their use. However, some practical books and plans that teach the sound principles of weight management are available. People who lose weight may have difficulty actually keeping it off, and it is important to use sound plans to encourage lifelong success.

Many weight-loss supplements are on the market, with most promising amazing results. Unfortunately, data do not support the efficacy of many products and limited research data are available on some of the others, so that no firm conclusions about their safety and efficacy can be made. Less is known about long-term safety.

The data available suggests that to lose weight and keep it off, the two key factors are controlled energy intake and regular physical activity. Losing and keeping off weight takes hard work and dedication—a message that consumers may not want to hear. People may want to purchase a magic pill and watch the pounds melt away. Obesity would not be the epidemic that it is today if losing and maintaining weight were as easy as some diets and supplements promise.

Section Four

Sport Performance Nutrition

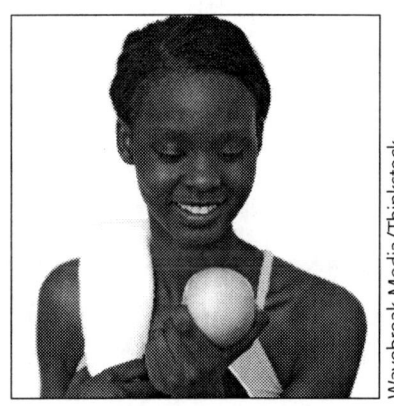

CHAPTER 10
SPORT DRINKS

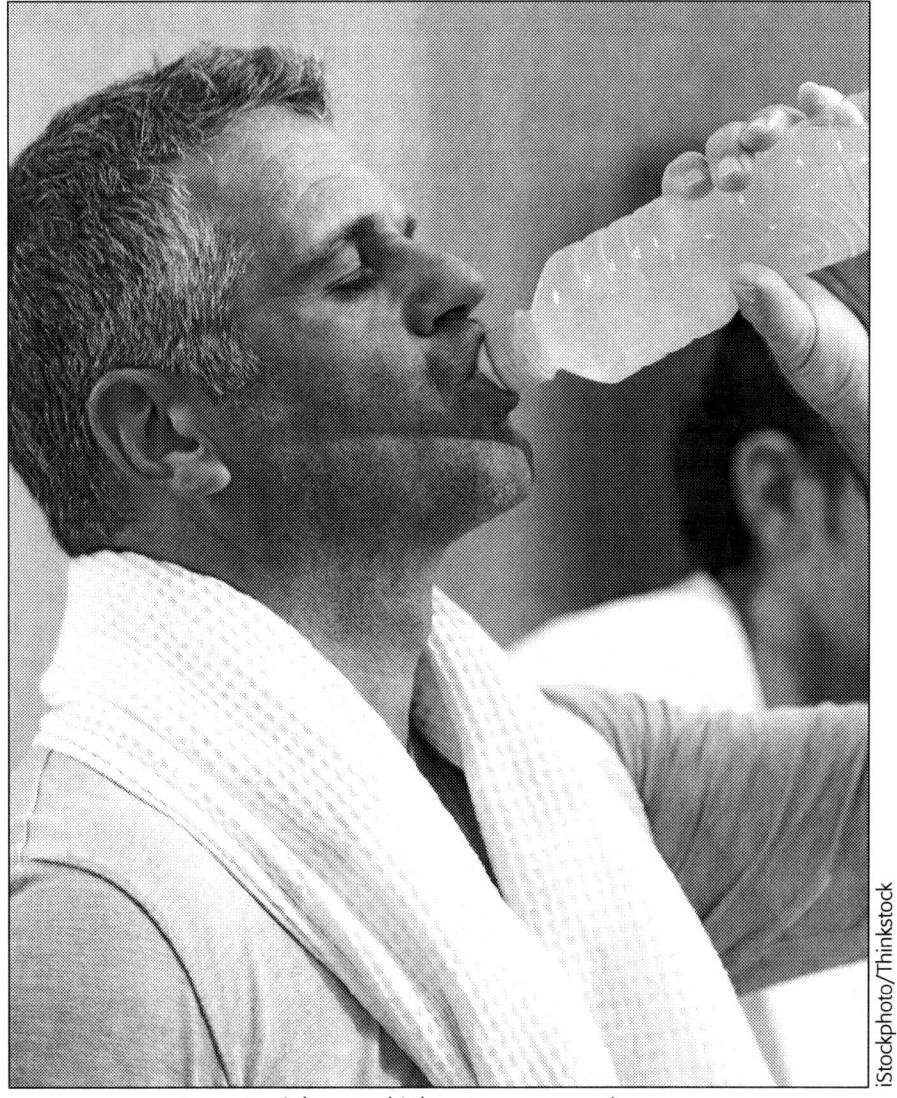

Commercial sport drinks are not a magic energy food, and often contain unhealthful ingredients.

Dehydration reduces your capacity for exercise and your tolerance of heat. Various advertisements for commercial sport drinks claim they prevent dehydration better than water. Is that so? Sport drink ads may state they replace electrolytes. What are electrolytes, and why and when do you need them? What else may be in these drinks? Are some of these drinks even healthful?

What Are Sport Drinks?

You lose water and salts in normal processes all day. You also burn carbohydrate for energy. You need to replace what you lose. Even though you can normally do so with regular healthful meals, commercial replacement drinks of all kinds have become a multi-billion-dollar industry. Just as worrisome, even if sugar water will extend endurance, it is increasingly recognized as junk food, and not healthful for the long term.

A major 2007 study by the World Cancer Research Fund made 10 recommendations for reducing risk of cancer, including getting exercise every day and drinking water rather than sugary drinks. Trendy sport and energy drinks add cost, plastic-bottle litter, and sometimes dyes, synthetic isolated vitamins, and questionable sweeteners. Increasingly, they contain stimulant compounds such as caffeine, guarana, ginseng, ephedra or ma huang. Use of stimulating compounds is linked to sleeplessness and increased nervousness and anxiety, and can become habit-forming. Drinks containing dyes, sweeteners, and stimulants are not a healthy choice for adults, and even less so for children and teens. Instead, you can easily make healthy whole-food sport drinks and vitamin water yourself for pennies.

You Get Thirsty Two Ways

One way you get thirsty is when you are low on water, called hypovolemic thirst. If you replace only water, your body sees that you have more fluid relative to electrolytes, because you have also lost electrolytes. Your body responds by "peeing" out some water to balance things. You may still be a bit low on water because of this response, even after drinking water, which is why it helps to get water from eating a piece of fruit. You replace a variety of needs through a whole food.

The second way you get thirsty is when you have a high-electrolyte blood content, regardless of your body's total water volume. This condition is called osmotic thirst. It is why salty things make you thirsty, even when you are drinking, and why bars serve salty finger food—to keep you drinking. Small amounts of sodium in electrolyte drinks stimulate your osmotic thirst, and then help you retain what you drink. It is why people drink more of these beverages than plain water, whether they need it or not.

What Is an Electrolyte?

An electrolyte is a substance that, when you dissolve it in liquid, becomes electrically conductive. Why does your body need an electric current? To transmit every signal for all the thousands of functions that nerves control to keep you alive, moving, and thinking, and to maintain an electrical potential across the membrane of every cell in your body, so that the cells can do their jobs.

No current flows through pure water. Dissolving even a trace of electrolytes in water makes water conductive. Electrolytes that are put into a liquid break up into ions. Ions are atoms or molecules with at least one or more fewer electrons than normal, giving them a positive or negative electric charge. Table salt, for example, becomes the positively charged sodium ion, and the negatively charged chloride ion. Both elements are principle ions in your body. In physiology, the ions themselves are called electrolytes. Salt itself is not an electrolyte, but in liquid it becomes the ions that are electrolytes.

The difference between current in electronic equipment and in your body is that electronic signals race through wire, passed by electrons, at up to half the speed of light, while in your body, nerve signals move through ions, thousands of times more slowly. Current in electronics uses electrons to pass the charge. The electrons themselves don't move far, but pass the charge along from one electron to the next like toppling dominoes. In your body, nerve signals move along dissolved ions. Like electrons, the ions themselves don't move far in the nerve, but propagate the signal by positive and negative ions switching places on either side of the nerve membrane. That exchange makes neighboring positive and negative ions want to switch places, too, in a continuing action called the action potential, until the signal is passed along the nerve. Then, the nerve ending uses a transmitter chemical to jump to the next nerve to start the signal traveling again, until the message is delivered.

Why Replace Electrolytes?

Losing some electrolytes through sweat is a good thing, to an extent. If you lost only water, your blood would become too concentrated with electrolytes. Even though you lose electrolytes, your body regulates the loss so you don't lose too much. When you sweat, you lose proportionately more water than minerals, leaving your blood slightly more concentrated than normal, or hypertonic. You can lose a substantial amount of electrolytes with prolonged sweating, creating a need for replacement. Without replacement, your electrolyte and fluid levels fall too low, and your ability to exercise decreases.

With extreme electrolyte loss during long exercise, and only water to drink without food to supply other nutrients, you may abnormally dilute your body fluids and cells, a condition called water intoxication. Effects range from weakness to convulsion and occasionally death. Water intoxication is also called hyponatremia, meaning low sodium in the blood. Cases are usually reported in hikers and distance runners who drink only large amounts of water and eat no food. Occasionally, serious cases of hyponatremia occur in infants swallowing pool water during parent-baby swimming lessons.

Your Body Regulates Electrolytes

You eat varying amounts of electrolytes in your food and drink, and lose varying amounts with exercise and daily activity. Your body ordinarily keeps levels of everything within narrow ranges, no matter how much you vary input and output.

Your body restricts electrolyte loss when your supply is low, and gets rid of excess when you eat or drink too much. When you are inactive, the major exit avenue for surplus electrolytes is urine and feces. When you are active and start sweating more, your body restricts the amount of electrolytes that exit with sweat, and secretes a hormone called aldosterone into your bloodstream to help your kidneys retain more sodium.

Most people in Western society eat many times more salt than their bodies require, sometimes in astounding quantities in fast foods, before they even pick up the saltshaker. When you eat more salt than you need, your body retains water to dilute the salt, and aldosterone secretion drops, encouraging your kidneys to excrete the excess.

"Salt-sensitive" people with high blood pressure need to restrict salt to allow them to lose the extra water that salt retains. Their blood pressure increases with salt intake. For the rest of the population, the kidneys tightly regulate output to get rid of excess electrolytes and water, or hang on to them, depending on what is needed at the time.

When Should You Replace Electrolytes?

Except for extreme endurance activities, you usually eat and drink more than enough electrolytes with your regular meals to keep you going. Ordinary recreational exercise does not deplete electrolytes enough to affect athletic ability or health. For that reason, after a one-hour bout of exercise, you don't ordinarily need to replace electrolytes immediately. It is also unnecessary to take extra electrolytes ahead of time to offset any loss predicted during your short bout of exercise. You don't lose enough to affect performance or cause fatigue. Unless you are in endurance races, or work long hours in hot environments with limited chance to eat and drink fluids other than water, health problems from electrolyte loss are unlikely.

Long-Term Effects

Commercial electrolytes drinks often contain refined sugar and other ingredients that are not healthful over the long term. Salt and sugar drinks can be helpful for specific uses: if a person is dangerously ill from a dehydrating disease such as cholera or dysentery, is suffering dehydration from prolonged vomiting, or has serious heat illness from lack of blood sugar and salt. For healthy athletes who are exercising, replacing blood sugar and salt helps performance and helps prevent heat injury. However, habitually consuming refined sugar is not healthful over the long term. Dyes and stimulants are linked with negative effect on emotional control. Isolated vitamins may also negatively affect health. Simple drinks you can make yourself, using ordinary, whole, healthful food, are a better choice.

How to Make Your Own Sport Drinks

You don't need to purchase commercial drinks. You can make your own healthier drink of various kinds, quickly and more cheaply. To make simple vitamin water:

- Put clean water in a blender.
- Add a few grapes with the skin and seeds, and blend well.

Grape skins and seeds have been found to contain cancer-fighting and other disease-fighting compounds. Think of the money you save by not buying expensive grapeseed oil products.

For a different light flavor, squeeze in fresh lemon. It helps keep the container cleaner, too. If you like tea, put a tea bag in the container. No need for hot water. To make different flavors, try a few strawberries with the green tops, watermelon with the seeds, or some raw sweet red pepper to make a variety of light, vitamin-water drinks.

Considerations for Sport Drinks

- You need to replace lost water and nutrients if you do endurance events lasting more than an hour or so, like marathons and triathlons.
- Consuming some food and water helps if you exercise in the heat for long periods.
- You do not need commercial or special sport-drink products. You can make your own from ordinary food and water.
- Be aware that commercial drinks promising energy may contain stimulant compounds. Habitual use can produce dependence, emotional change, sleeplessness, and unsafe interactions with common prescription and other drugs. Other common effects include feeling nervous with the consumption of the drinks and unwell without it.

Healthier Containers

Commercially bottled fitness water and drinks may not be healthful, from the drink inside to the container they come in. Plastic containers may leach chemicals into the drink they hold, and the bottling, transport, and disposal all seriously weaken environmental fitness—and ultimately your own. The plastic water bottle manufacturing process requires 1.5 million barrels of crude oil a year. Bottling and shipping water produced more than 2.5 million tons of carbon dioxide in 2006. When you carry your homemade fitness drinks and water with you, use safe, non-plastic bottles. Instead of spending money on bottled water, get a water filter for your tap water. Research demonstrates that the water supply increasingly contains medical drugs excreted by the users and other chemicals that constitute a "body burden" of compounds with potential health effects.

Healthier Sport and Energy Drink Choices

Your health benefits from good hydration. During extended intense exercise, you can replace needed electrolyte, carbohydrate, and protein with ordinary food or simple homemade drinks. Commercial sport drinks are not a magic energy food, and often contain unhealthful ingredients. You can easily make your own healthier sport drinks. Don't worry that you must eat engineered commercial products or you can't win. You can win better in the long run without them.

Why You Get Dehydrated From Drinking Seawater

Sea-going birds—such as penguins, seagulls, petrels, and albatross—can drink seawater. Special glands in their heads excrete excess salt. Humans also have to get rid of the extra salt in seawater because the amount is just too much for your system, yet you have no salt-excreting glands. Your blood is not similar in composition to seawater (contrary to popular belief). Your blood is several times more dilute. If your blood were like seawater, you could safely drink seawater, which is not the case. In the process of excreting the excess salt in salt water, the human kidney draws water from the body's supply, a process so dehydrating that if seawater were the only fluid replacement available, you could die of thirst faster if you drank seawater than if you didn't.

CHAPTER 11
PERFORMANCE-ENHANCING FOODS

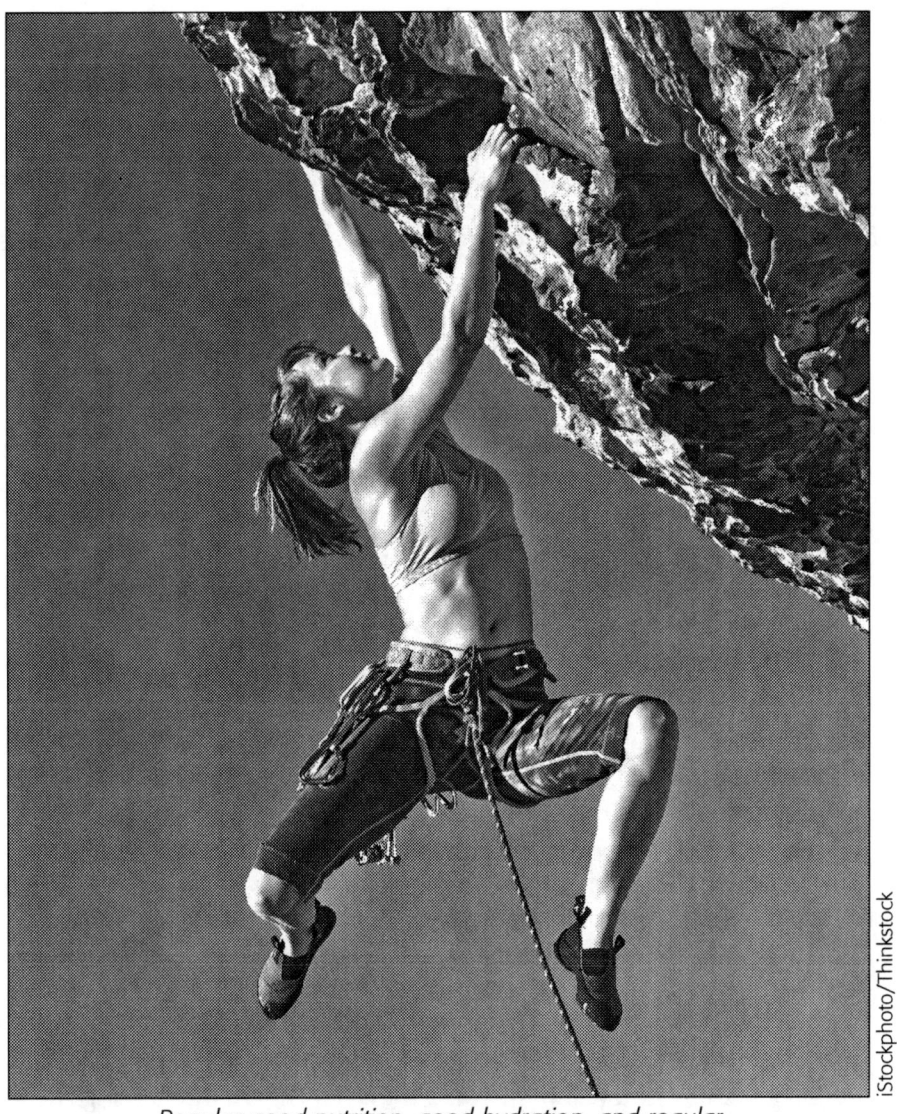

Regular good nutrition, good hydration, and regular exercise (not supplements) give true athletic advantage.

The search for a personal edge that you can eat is a common one. Hundreds of years ago, Aztec warriors ate the hearts of fearless enemies, believing it would increase their own bravery. To prepare for battle, the Inca Indians chewed coca leaves, and Berserkers ate muscaria mushrooms, which made them seem and act wild. Norsemen drank the milk of Arctic reindeer in heat. In the Middle Ages, Dervishes whirled longer using coffee. Sigmund Freud used cocaine. Today, South American Indians know chewing coca leaves reduces hunger and fatigue. In the Middle East, *khat* leaves are chewed for similar effect. Betel nuts are chewed in Asia and the South Pacific Islands, and the kola nut in the Sudan. Some people take diet pills, eat protein supplements, use steroids, drink coffee, or try preparations with labels promising everything from muscle growth to energetic hair.

What Is an Ergogenic Aid?

Substances and practices that help physical performance are sometimes called ergogenic aids. An *erg* is a unit of work. The word "energy" contains the erg root and means the ability to do work. The suffix *-gen* means "producing" or "generating." Putting them together forms the word "ergogenic" and refers to things used and, not incidentally, believed to enhance physical performance. Not everything claiming to be ergogenic is really ergogenic.

Some ergogenic aids are psychological, such as mental rehearsal, confidence training, and good-luck charms. Some are physical, such as hard exercise, lifting weights, or training at altitude. Nutritional ergogenic aids include an assortment of drugs, supplements, and food concoctions. Some are hokum—many products on the market claiming to be ergogenic have no ergogenic properties. Others work well enough to be banned by athletic associations and Olympic committees. Certain products work, but are unhealthful or addictive.

Why Do People Use Ergogenic Aids?

Would you pay to eat a product called "This Won't Work," or would you prefer "Beautiful Body For Certain"? Many products are sold through clever advertising and false hope. Product names are not required by law to do what they imply, allowing ads to combine suggestive words like *power, energy, natural, super, organic, health,* and *mega* on their labels. Who could think a vitamin named Ener-B® didn't have anything to do with feeling energetic? Ads targeting the serious bodybuilder market suggest anabolic steroid capability with names incorporating word segments like *ana, testo,* and *bolic,* even if they do not have those components. Product promotions may include quotes from flawed studies in obscure or faux journals. The Food and Drug Administration (FDA) does not currently require testing these products for proof of efficacy. An athlete may work and slave, eat low fat, train diligently, but then attribute all gains to a capsule or pill, and go on to promote the product through testimonials.

Another reason people use certain substances is that some of the potions work to various degrees. Cardiac relaxants can improve aim in target shooting. Stimulants boost speed and endurance. Other substances increase muscle mass.

Many stimulant preparations are sold as "natural" and "herbal," which does not mean they are harmless or non-addictive. Nicotine, for example, is a naturally occurring plant substance. Do not buy stimulants thinking they will have no problems because they are labeled "natural." Herbal medicines are not necessarily safer or more natural than any other pill or medicine. Dependence on Eastern medicine is no different than dependence on Western pills. Check to see if you are relying on products instead of making healthy lifestyle changes. You could have energy, weight loss, and increased physical abilities by exercising more, eating better, and stopping smoking, without spending on dubious pills.

> Natural" and "herbal" do not mean harmless or non-addictive.

Methylxanthene Stimulants

Coffee

Few people who drink coffee or cola drinks consider themselves drug users. These drinks contain caffeine, the most commonly used stimulant drug in the world. Other people shun caffeine, and instead take "natural" stimulant herbs. Caffeine is no less "natural" than any health food herb. They can all have the same unwanted effects.

The effect of caffeine after eating berries and seeds containing it was probably discovered in the Stone Age. It has been widely used ever since. Caffeine can extend endurance, and it is banned in high concentrations by the International Olympic Committee for that reason. A big rage for caffeine as an ergogenic aid may have begun in 1978 when exercise physiologist David Costil, told *Runner's World* magazine that caffeine could improve marathon times. According to Professor of Medicine Randy Eichner, "This led to long coffee lines at big marathons, followed by long potty lines."

How caffeine helps is still studied and debated. Caffeine is thought to help endurance by directly stimulating your central nervous system, decreasing your perception of effort, helping your body save some fuel called glycogen, and possibly improving your use of fat as fuel. More recently, caffeine is thought to help short-term activity (so brief that your body has no time to use either glycogen or fat) possibly by increasing recruitment of more of your muscle fibers and/or directly increasing their resistance to fatigue. Coffee itself may have antioxidant properties.

Reactions to caffeine vary and may change throughout your lifetime. Effects may be partly genetically based, and partly due to how much you eat with it, time of day, how much you are accustomed to, and other interactions. For most people, nervousness, increased urine production, and heartbeat irregularities begin after one cup, and increase with dosage, with increasing tendency to irregular heart rhythms from caffeine as you get older. Many commercially sold preparations claiming energy effects from herbs contain caffeine or caffeine-like substances.

The body becomes accustomed to regular caffeine intake. Regular drinkers frequently experience withdrawal symptoms of headache, irritability, and weariness as soon as missing even a single expected dose. If you are a coffee drinker, try to keep use low to moderate.

Theobromine

Cocoa, gotukola nut, and several other foodstuffs contain theobromine, among other substances. Theobromine stimulates the nervous system, opens airways, and increases heart rate, but less intensely than caffeine. Theobromine is used in certain medicines and advertised in some supplements promising energy. Eating real unsweetened cocoa is a healthful source of theobromine and several healthful antioxidants and other compounds. Dark chocolate has more theobromine than lighter chocolate, with flavonoids and phenolics, which are plant substances that are good for the heart. Candy and chocolate product manufacturers may use a process called Dutching (or Dutch process) to remove flavonols, polyphenols, and other healthful compounds in cocoa, because of their bitter taste, and often add fat and sugar, which are harmful to the heart and arteries. Instead of buying cocoa made into unhealthful chocolate candy, look for powdered unsweetened, non-alkalized (non-Dutched) cocoa or unsweetened baking squares. It can be found easily in the grocery baking section. Add to blender drinks, baking, and desserts. For some people who get a kind of vascular headache called migraine, chocolate may trigger the headache. They do better not to eat chocolate.

Sympathomimetic Stimulants

Part of your nervous system increases heart rate and constricts blood vessels, getting you "ready to go." That part of your nervous system is called the sympathetic nervous system. Substances with properties that mimic your sympathetic nervous system are called sympathomimetic. Three examples are amphetamines, cocaine, and ma huang. Not everything that is a central nervous system stimulant is sympathomimetic (for example, caffeine and nicotine). People use sympathomimetics because they inhibit fatigue and appetite. Overstimulation and addiction are common, resulting in various effects that are not healthy. Many products sold as "health" and energy food have stimulant compounds that have unhealthful, even dangerous effects, especially when combined with other stimulating compounds, coffee, many prescription medicines, cold medicines, and various performance-enhancing substances.

Amphetamines

Amphetamines are addictive stimulants. Amphetamines became popular as "pep pills," athletic enhancers, anti-depressants, and diet pills because they mask tiredness, sadness, and hunger. Amphetamines were given to military forces during World War II to delay fatigue, even mixed with chocolate, called "flier's chocolate" and "tanker's chocolate." A large post-war health epidemic followed. Methamphetamine, or meth, is an amphetamine prone to abuse and addiction. A large population, including young children, has become addicted from wide use in medical prescriptions. Dangerous effects have been dismissed as "side effects."

Amphetamine users may experience abnormally high or irregular heart rates, raised blood pressure, and sometimes mental states resembling paranoid schizophrenia. Abdominal cramps, incoordination, dizziness, dry mouth, nausea, and vomiting may accompany initial use. Some people experience unusual effects on their blood cells. Stimulants like amphetamines, ephedra, and Ritalin® raise risk of heart trouble. Amphetamines constrict the arterioles of the skin (small, end branches of skin arteries), increasing risk of overheating. Deaths in endurance competitions in the heat have been connected to amphetamine use.

Amphetamines usually addict their user physically and psychologically. Abusers can gradually increase their doses from 10 to 1,000 times to retain the initial effects. Withdrawal brings uncomfortable rebound symptoms of hunger and weakness. Users are prone to unhealthful actions to procure more amphetamines to stop the withdrawal pain.

For solving problems in concentration and mood, amphetamines are not a healthy practice. For weight control, diet pills undermine sound nutrition and allow the user to ignore the requirement of exercise in fat reduction, predisposing the user to serious health consequences. Newer diet pills replacing the older amphetamine types still require extreme caution. Moreover, after two to three weeks, diet pills begin losing effectiveness.

What is an effective substitute for amphetamine drugs? Exercise. Exercise increases feelings of energy and happiness, and offsets food calories for weight control.

Cocaine

Cocaine enhances physical performance, with an unhealthy price. Cocaine is sympathomimetic. Your nerve endings release nerve transmission chemicals called catecholamines across a space, called a synapse, to the next nerve ending. After they have done their job to transmit their signal, you have to get the catecholamine back out of the synapse so it doesn't keep signaling and signaling. Several normal mechanisms accomplish that task, including gathering the catecholamine back up into storage areas in the nerve endings, ready for more signaling at another time. Cocaine blocks this reuptake, prolonging the effects of released catecholamines. For this reason, you get so much signaling with cocaine—lots of it. Signaling in some areas of your brain feels good.

As with other central-nervous-system stimulants, the extra signaling increases heart rate and muscle contraction, allowing more physical work, and making you feel "geared up" to do that work. Signaling to your heart and blood vessels, from the catecholamine called norepinephrine, raises blood pressure and increases abnormal heartbeats. Too much of this signaling to the heart can cause a sudden, sometimes fatal, heart attack. Surviving that situation, the problem with not taking up your catecholamines again for reuse means that you can run out. Running out of your catecholamine stores leads to severe depression (the cocaine crash).

> Many health foods and herbal remedies sold as "pick-me-ups," athletic enhancers, and weight-loss aids contain various central nervous system stimulants.

Other Stimulants

Ginseng

Herbal energy potions claiming that they are caffeine-free does not necessarily mean they are free of side effects or are healthy for you. Ginseng is an example. Because of ginseng's stimulant effects, it is popularly used for a variety of health problems and for a general "pick-me-up." Ginseng is used in pills, teas, sodas, candies, and drinks. Ginseng can affect glucose metabolism and raise heart rate and blood pressure. If you overmedicate yourself with ginseng, you can wind up with diarrhea, nervousness, skin rashes, and insomnia. Most symptoms will disappear when use is reduced or discontinued. It doesn't mean ginseng is bad; just that it is not harmless. It has effects, which is why people take it.

Most of the biological effects of ginseng come from ginsenosides. Investigations have found that content varies greatly, with some ginseng preparations containing no ginsenosides at all. Laws do not require uniformity or even labeling to identify content.

As with other stimulant use, take a look at your health habits to find out why you want stimulants. Taking them can produce a vicious cycle of dependence and fatigue without them, and a cycle of being too stimulated to sleep well at night, creating daytime fatigue. Poor eating habits, too much simple sugar, not enough exercise, and too much time spent indoors contribute to general malaise. Don't use stimulants to combat poor habits. Use healthy ways to give you energy. Herb stimulants are drugs the same as any other potions and pills.

Steroids and Steroid Substitutes

Anabolic Steroids

The word "anabolic" means promoting tissue growth. Not all steroids are anabolic. The anti-inflammatories cortisone and prednisone are steroids, and they are not anabolic. They do not stimulate growth. Neither does Vitamin D, another steroid that is not an anabolic steroid.

Anabolic steroids are controlled substances. They are prescription oral and/or injectable drugs that have anabolic and masculinizing or androgenic effects. They are often used to fatten cattle to enhance market price. A large problem of steroid use exists in school-age and older athletes wanting physical gains at any price. A large black market exists for prescription medical and veterinary anabolic steroids. Adverse physical and emotional side effects of anabolic steroids include high blood pressure, elevated "bad" cholesterol (LDL), liver and kidney damage, greater risk of heart and vascular disease, and volatile, aggressive, and recklessly uncontrolled behaviors. Long-term use reduces your own body's production of male hormones. Male genitalia can shrink. Some steroids increase female hormones, causing men's breasts to grow. Users trying to avoid these side effects add use of anti-estrogen drugs, which have their own side effects. Users may not be aware that their personality is changing. Side effects are common and incompatible with physical and emotional health. Don't let your ego get in the way of your health. You can be a bigger, more powerful person by giving the money spent on self-indulgent drug use to the poor and being a role model for honest exercise. Exercise increases your body's production of anabolic hormones without the side effects. Decreases in normal body levels with aging can be offset by healthy fun exercise.

Growth Hormone

Growth hormone is naturally made in the pituitary gland of your brain. It does several things, including stimulating protein to make muscle. Injections of synthetic growth hormone are used by bodybuilders and athletes hoping for strength and size increase and by actors and models hoping to look more muscular and lean. Some cosmetic procedure doctors promote it as a drug against various signs of aging. Growth hormone use is not yet detectable by drug testing. The American College of Sports Medicine (ACSM) strongly advises against supplemental growth hormone for athletic enhancement because of ethical and physical problems.

In children, one function of growth hormone is to stimulate bone lengthening. When the pituitary doesn't produce enough, children don't grow enough, causing one form of dwarfism. Occasionally, with too much hormone, a child can grow to a giant. An adult taking growth hormone after bone maturation will not increase long bone length, so cannot get taller. Instead the forehead, hands, feet, and jaw may elongate.

Human growth hormone for medical use was originally extracted from the human pituitary glands of cadavers and abbreviated "hGH." By 1985, concerns about transmitting incurable fatal brain diseases like Creutzfeldt-Jakob Disease led to replacing pituitary-derived hGH with synthetic growth hormone. The injectable form is not human growth hormone (made from humans), but synthetic, which has a different name.

Human growth hormone (hGH) is no longer used in medicine or sport doping. Instead, biosynthetic human growth hormone is used, called recombinant human growth hormone (rhGH), somatropin, somatotropin, or somatotrophin (somatotrophs are the pituitary cells where the human form is made). Even if products are marked "hGH," they would contain no growth hormone (and you would not want them to). The underground market of performance-enhancing drugs is known for having many fake (counterfeit) drugs for sale, including fake growth hormone.

Growth hormone "doping" is expensive, and must be done for a long time before results occur. For bigger results, some bodybuilders and athletes combine, or "stack," growth hormones with anabolic steroids (bodybuilding hormones). Some users add the dangerous practice of injecting insulin in combination with growth hormone (and/or steroids) for bigger muscles, more veins showing, and the appearance of exceptionally thin skin, looking as if shrink-wrapped over the muscle (believed a desirable look by some people). Insulin doping can cause serious, long-term illnesses.

Problems from growth hormone doping can include joint pain, wrist pain, carpal tunnel syndrome, joint swelling, facial swelling, facial elongation, and increased blood pressure. Using large doses can decrease thyroid function and increase risk of diabetes. Sadly, users may think these effects are signs of aging, so they take more growth hormone believing it will stop this "aging." If the user already has cancer, it can increase growth of the tumor.

Growth hormone is naturally produced in your body throughout your life. Older people produce less growth hormone, but they still produce it. Some advertising for GH tries to persuade its targets that older people are somehow at a disadvantage without a lot. Remember that older people (above the age range of puberty) need less because they are not growing, although they still need enough for strength and tissue repair. Aging alone is not what makes you not have enough growth hormone. Four main factors reduce your body's growth-hormone levels:

- *Lack of exercise.* Without exercise, your muscles, bones, and other tissues have no reason to rebuild; you aren't using them, after all.
- *High blood sugar from dietary sources* (e.g., eating too much, eating too often, eating without enough exercise to use the blood sugar, and eating junk food).
- *Too much growth hormone.* Your body reduces its growth hormone levels if it already has too much. Growth hormone stimulates your liver and other tissues to secrete "insulin-like growth factor-I" (IGF-I), which is the real factor behind most of the effects of growth hormone. Having high blood levels of IGF-I decreases secretion of growth hormone as a normal regulatory function.

- *Ongoing dosage with anti-inflammatory and immune-suppressive medicines called glucocorticoids* (such as prednisone, dexamethasone, and hydrocortisone). People taking these medicines for injuries and pain should keep in mind that ongoing dosage can lead to osteoporosis, muscle weakness, delayed wound healing, and increased infection risk.

How do you get more natural growth hormone in healthy amounts without side effects? Three main agents stimulate GH secretion in your body:

- *Exercise.* Getting exercise in healthful ways, described throughout this book, boosts GH at all ages.
- *Deep sleep.* With good exercise, you will sleep well at night, too.
- *Low levels of sugar in your blood.* It is shown that both high fat and high refined-sugar diets increase blood sugar. It is not rocket science to eat less junk and more fruit and vegetables to be healthier and to lower high blood sugar. Taking supplemental GH in adults may irreversibly increase growth of the jaw, forehead, hands, and feet, even in cases where it does not increase strength. It may also increase risk of diabetes, high blood pressure, and heart problems.

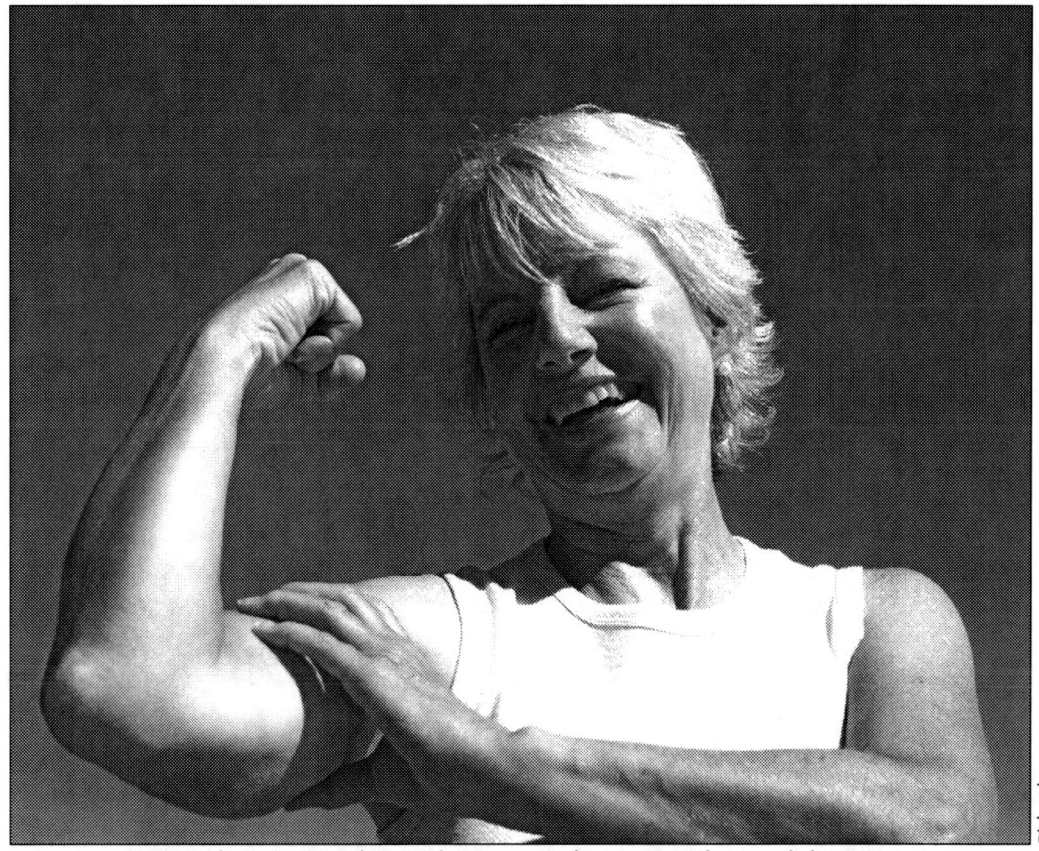

Aging alone is not what makes you not have enough growth hormone.

Compounds supposedly having GH-releasing potential sell briskly in health-food stores and gyms. Ornithine and sapogenin are two growth hormone hopefuls that fall short. Ornithine is often packaged in 250mg capsules, although the effective dose is far higher. Sapogens are derived from plants found in desert regions. Your body will excrete them without making any GH. If you want results similar to taking growth hormone, but in a natural, safe, and inexpensive manner without side effects, vigorous exercise does that.

Anabolic Activators, Multipacs, and Enhancers

Packs of food elements are usually labeled with the suggestive name "anabolic." They have no special muscle-building abilities, and contain nothing that is not available in regular food. They are not anabolic steroids or steroid substitutes, except by name, and no law currently prevents anyone from selling you potions called steroid substitutes, even if they have no anabolic steroid effect. The name "steroid substitute" means only that advertisers would like you to buy their products instead of steroids, not necessarily that the product works like steroids do. The use of the word "anabolic" could technically mean that, since some of these supplements have so many calories, they do promote tissue growth—of fat—the same way any other high-calorie food does.

"Women's" Sport Supplements

A large and unfortunate industry exists of convincing people they need to spend money on separate sport and health supplements for women. Estrogenic, or estrogen-promoting, supplements are easily overconsumed and are increasingly documented to contribute to estrogen-dependent tumors such as fibroids, cystic ovary, breast cysts, and endometriosis.

A partial list of estrogenic products includes unfermented soy, primrose oil, chasteberry, kudzu, black cohosh, St. John's Wort, dong quai, pennyroyal, flax seeds, burdock root. More are absorbed through the skin in lotions and oils containing lavender, clary sage, high amounts of tea-tree oil, and from hair products and shampoos with hormone containing placenta and estrogen or its precursors.

Hundreds of thousands of women annually have needless, serious, and painful surgery for conditions they might alleviate by avoiding overloading on estrogenic foods and the numerous "women's" supplements sold in "health" food stores.

Protein

The most common belief about protein supplementation is that eating more protein will build bigger muscles. It won't. Consider the following: Protein enters into thousands of body functions besides muscle assembly. Eating more protein will not automatically increase all those functions. Protein builds skin, enters into the reactions that create the pigment in your skin, and is a building block for the smooth muscle in your blood vessels. Extra protein doesn't grow more skin, make you turn brown, or make your blood vessels more muscular.

> Protein has many functions in your body besides growing muscles. Eating more protein does not increase any of those functions in speed or amount. For example, protein is involved in pigmenting your skin, but eating extra protein does not darken your skin.

Do You Need More Protein When Active?

Studies find that for a brief time after beginning an exercise program, your body's protein balance falls, then restores to previous levels. The need to increase protein (over the recommended minimum) may be brief and mild. Most people routinely eat more protein than the required recommended daily allowance (RDA). Because of all they already eat, any increased intake in meals or supplements is often unnecessary.

> A high-protein meat dinner can keep you from sleeping well. Get legume- and vegetable-based protein meals throughout the day, and most of your protein at breakfast and lunch.

You can't store protein the way you can store fat and, to a lesser extent, carbohydrate. Whenever you eat more protein than you need on any given day, most will convert to fat, and you will excrete the rest, a process requiring water. In high amounts, dietary protein contributes to dehydration and loss of calcium.

For the average inactive person, the minimum RDA for protein is 0.8 grams for every kilogram of body weight. A kilogram is about 2.2 pounds, making your minimum requirement less than half a gram of protein for every pound you weigh. Protein requirement for a 180-pound (82 kilogram) person varies around 65 grams per day, or about 2 ounces. A 130-pound person (59 kilograms) meets minimum requirements with less than 50 grams.

An active athlete may need at least 1 gram per kilogram of body weight. Muscle magazines often state that you need a gram of protein or more per pound of body weight. This amount does not seem to be the case, and has not been shown to have any effect on muscle building. Strength athletes usually need less protein than endurance athletes. Endurance athletes need a bit more protein, as they burn more calories. Muscle requires little protein for growth. For active people, carbohydrate supplementation seems to be more important and contributes more to muscle building.

> You need a certain amount of protein every day. You may need more than that amount when you are active. The average person already eats more protein than required and so has no need to supplement.

Not All Protein Sources Are Healthful

Check supplement protein powders for fillers, dyes, sweeteners, thickeners, and hidden stimulants to give a false good feeling or weight loss in unhealthful manner. Dairy and whey products have many of the unhealthful components of dairy, compounded by drying, processing, and concentrating them. Products with soy are usually unfermented soy. Unfermented soy contains enzyme inhibitors (which block digestion), goitrogens (which inhibit thyroid function), phytic acid (which blocks minerals like zinc and calcium), and estrogen-promoting compounds. Anyone with a tendency toward estrogen-dependent tumors or cancer, fibroids, cystic ovary or breast, or endometriosis should avoid unfermented soy. In general, vegetable, non-soy sources of protein from real whole food are best.

In a study published in the *European Journal of Clinical Nutrition* (November 29, 2006), researchers found that eating diets of low carbohydrate and high protein was associated with "increased mortality and risk of cancer." Another study, published in the *American Journal of Clinical Nutrition* (December 2006), concluded that a low-protein diet may protect against certain cancers. Other research published in 2007 from the University of Leeds found that those with the highest intake of red meat, the equivalent to one portion a day (more than 57 grams), run a 56 percent greater risk of breast cancer than those who eat none. Women who eat the most processed meat—such as bacon, sausages, or ham—run a 64 percent greater risk of breast cancer than those women who eat none. Large studies in England and Germany found a 40 percent lower risk of many kinds of cancer in vegetarians, both men and women, compared to meat eaters.

Good quality protein is available without meat, dairy, or supplement powders. Try beans, peas, lentils, sesame seeds, oats, brown rice, nuts, chickpeas, muesli, seaweed, kelp, brewers yeast, hummus, tahini, and spirulina. These foods have protein, antioxidants, many nutrients, and fiber.

It is not true that you need to carefully mix specific foods in each meal to get complete proteins from vegetables, grains, and legumes. Proteins combine on their own in the body over the day of eating a variety. It is another food myth that you must avoid eating protein with starch (carbohydrate), or not eat one food group in combination with others. Nutrients usually work better together.

You can build much strength and muscle without eating any supplements or high protein diets. Save your money. Just do honest exercise in healthy ways.

Carbohydrate

Carbohydrate provides energy for activities. Carbohydrate is so important that your body stores it, mostly in your muscles and liver in a form called glycogen. The larger your stores, the longer you can exercise before you fatigue, depending on your physical fitness. You increase your body carbohydrate stores when you exercise regularly and eat regular meals with (healthful) carbohydrate.

Many commercial energy bars, mixes, and drinks are little more than unhealthful candy, with refined sugar, fillers, dyes, hydrolyzed proteins, unhealthy fats, and some synthetic vitamins. Eating them does not make you healthy just because they have the words "natural," "healthy," "vitamins," or "exercise" on the label. You would get more vitamins and health from eating a pear and some walnuts. Any product that contains high fructose corn syrup is not something you need to eat. Processed packaged sport supplement foods cost far more than the ingredients, and you can get healthier ingredients at a lower cost, and just as easily to make your own without commercial sport powders, bars, drinks, and other preparations.

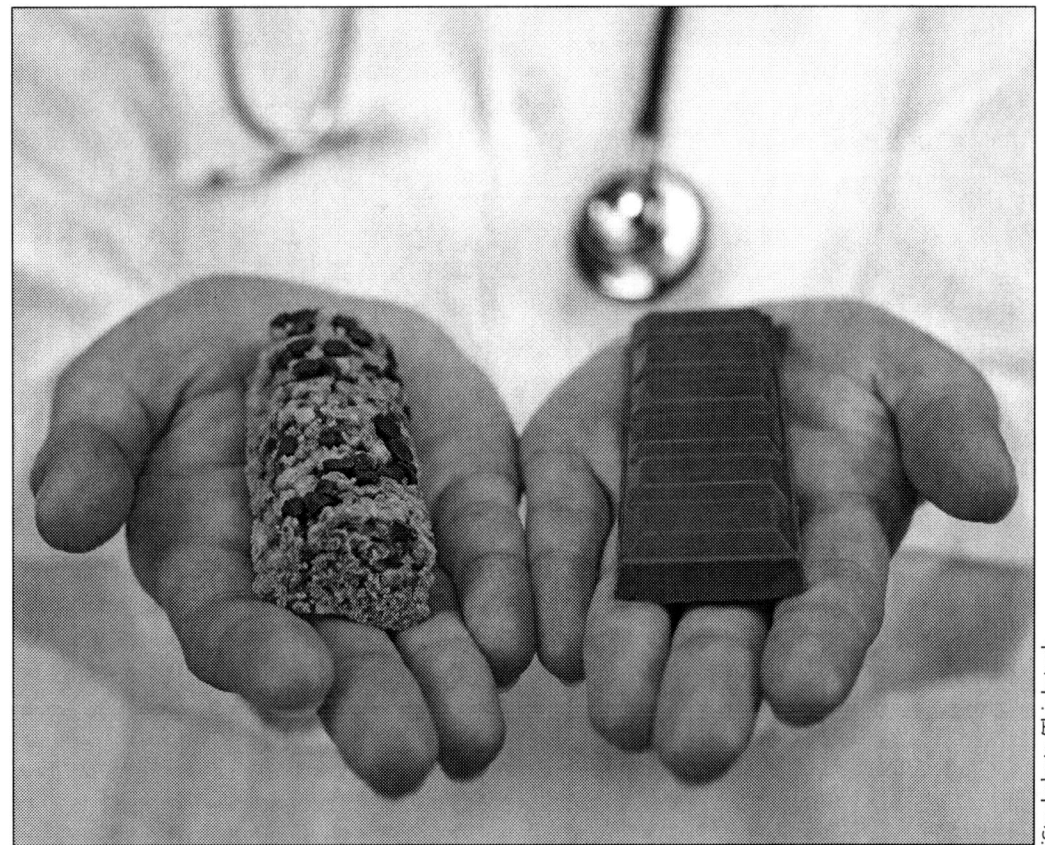

Many commercial energy bars, mixes, and drinks are little more than unhealthful candy, with refined sugar, fillers, dyes, hydrolyzed proteins, unhealthy fats, and some synthetic vitamins.

Because athletes exercising at high intensities for long periods can delay fatigue and, therefore, work longer and harder with added carbohydrates, misunderstandings result. Taking carbohydrate drinks and preparations will not transform you into a better athlete. Your ability to do submaximal exercise like recreational running, swimming, biking, dancing, walking, skating, and so on, does not improve from any particular food or drink. Moreover, drinking sugar water is not fitness or health.

Carbohydrate Loader and Replacement Drinks

Carbohydrate loader drinks have a higher carbohydrate content than regular electrolyte-replacer drinks for intense, long-duration exercise. "Energy food" technically means it has calories. Extra calories alone will not enable you to build muscle or win a race. Carbohydrate loader drinks are not magic energy elixirs. They won't give you a performance edge if taken before or during exercise much shorter than an hour or so, like an aerobics class, a half hour to an hour of cycling, skiing, or basketball, or even a 6- to 10-kilometer jog. Athletes generally have enough of their own stored carbohydrate, called glycogen, to last about an hour to 90 minutes.

Carbohydrate replacement drinks have a higher carbohydrate content than the loader drinks. Long, intense exercise depletes glycogen, an important fuel. You need to replace glycogen soon after exercise. If you don't, your body can't make enough glycogen to replace the loss. Your muscle and liver reserves remain low even days later, limiting further exercise ability.

The first 30 minutes after hard exercise are crucial to the major restocking. Your muscles can restore more total carbohydrate if you begin to eat or drink carbohydrates within 30 minutes after hard exercise. The next two hours are the second important stage. You benefit by eating complex carbohydrate food such as fruit, sweet potato, or a homemade drink recipe as soon after exercise as you can.

Drinks With "Buzz"

Packaged "health" and "sport" drinks may contain stimulants of many kinds: ginseng, ma huang, guarana, ephedra, caffeine and its variants, and others. These products are advertised as "energy" drinks. Check the label. You don't need them to exercise or lose weight. A cycle starts of needing the product to avoid feeling weary and headachy. Nervousness, anxiety, inability to concentrate by day and sleep at night, and irregular heartbeats can occur. Mixing these products with energy pills, diet pills, coffee and espresso, and other pills and medicines, can produce effects even more serious.

Users with uncomfortable effects may add over-the-counter or prescription medicines to try to stop those effects. That approach is not health. The practice of regularly taking stimulant drinks and products is a foolhardy one to become accustomed to, building cycles of inability to focus, exercise, or feel well without them, and varying degrees of agitation with them, sleep difficulties, and various cardiovascular risks.

> If amphetamines and cigarettes were discovered today, they would probably be in stores advertised as "wonder energy enhancers" and "natural" diet aids. Remember that they once were promoted that way with devastating health effects. Compare that when spending money on other commercial products for "energy."

Creatine

Chapter 3 explains how you use a molecule called ATP to fuel short, hard activity. As quickly as you use ATP, you rebuild it for more activity using creatine phosphate that you store, mostly in your muscles. You can't store much, only enough for 8 to 10 seconds of intense activity, like a 100-meter dash. When you run low, you shift to another energy system at lower intensity. The hope of supplemental creatine to fuel intense short efforts is behind sales of creatine as a supplement.

Creatine monohydrate is a synthetic of the creatine phosphate you make in your body. Not everyone can absorb it, which may be why some people find results using it and others don't. Advice to eat lots of steak and pork, which contain creatine, doesn't work (for you or the pig). Once you cook meat, the creatine denatures (changes permanently), so you can't use it. Harming your arteries with high-meat meals won't help athletic ability, either. You don't need to eat creatine directly because your body makes what you need from balanced meals, including vegetarian meals. Ergogenic effect of creatine supplementation seems to be counteracted by caffeine. One thing known to work well is to get in better shape. Good aerobic ability increases your ability to store the creatine that you make and use it to rebuild your energy stores. Even after years of inquiry, the USDA issued an advisory statement saying more is unknown than known about creatine side effects over the long term, and that adverse effects may result on your kidneys and liver.

Androstenedione (Andro)

"Andro" is another expensive "health food store" supplement. You make it in your own body out of DHEA. People buy it because androstenedione breaks down to testosterone, a male hormone. However, another hormone that androstenedione makes is estrogen. Body chemistry is more complicated than "andro makes muscles because it makes testosterone." Your body is smart. If it has too much of a substance, it will try to reduce the excess. Andro supplements can increase urinary levels—not because more hormone is in your body, but because your body is getting rid of the extra. Sometimes, your body will stop producing its own testosterone if it intakes too much, making you more deficient than when you started. Sometimes, andro supplements have other elements not on the label that can cause a positive drug test for banned substances.

Reports from gyms and androstenedione manufacturers state that andro always greatly helps athletic ability. Carefully done studies in real labs don't always find that it increases lean body mass, strength, or testosterone levels in healthy adult men. Some studies show increased strength, but only the same amount of strength as a control group who also exercised hard but didn't supplement with andro. Great changes into a muscular athlete don't happen from pills alone. Although andro is available over the counter, its use is banned by athletic bodies because of harmful side effects and ethical issues.

Vitamins

Many people regard vitamins as ergogenic aids. No scientific evidence supports vitamin supplementation as ergogenic. Unless you have a nutritional deficiency, increasing your intake will not improve physical ability.

Vitamins have no calories, so by definition they furnish no energy. Vitamins are often advertised as giving energy, even labeled with suggestive names like "Ener-B." Unless your fatigue relates to a deficiency, they will not make you energetic.

> **Vitamin B12 has been called the least likely vitamin to affect sport performance and the most likely to be abused for nonexistent ergogenic effects.**

Taking too many vitamins can be unhealthy. Some vitamins are fat-soluble. With repeated overdosing, they can accumulate in your body to toxic levels. Other vitamins are water-soluble and you excrete them, but can still have side effects with long-term overdose. Vitamins do not work in isolation. Studies find unhealthful effects of taking vitamin supplements, with some studies showing increased risk of cancer. It is better to get vitamins from whole foods where they exist along with many other compounds they need to work with that cannot be isolated into pills

Minerals

Like vitamins, minerals have no calories and no known ergogenic effects. Deficiencies may result in weaknesses, but taking amounts above your needs will not improve your physical fitness. Even so, many have been advertised with claims of ergogenic effects.

Boron is one of several minerals misrepresented as an ergogenic aid. A widely misquoted study found low dietary boron decreased testosterone in postmenopausal women. Levels rose when the deficiency was corrected. From that misquoted study came claims of boron as helpful to athletes to increase their testosterone levels, with "studies" seeming to back up those claims. Although problems stem from nutrient deficiency, no evidence suggests that extra boron elevates testosterone. Large doses are toxic. Boron is an ultra-trace mineral. You need only tiny amounts and can get them from fruits, vegetables, nuts, and legumes.

Chromium (including chromium picolinate) and vanadium are ultra-trace minerals in the diet that have been advertised as ergogenic. If a deficiency exists, the benefit of supplementation is to correct the deficiency. No good evidence suggests that they alter your body composition or enhance athletic ability to any extent that it matters to most exercisers.

Carnitine

The excitement over carnitine began when the Italian soccer team won a title while taking carnitine. The team did many other things besides taking carnitine, such as train at high levels. No specific evidence shows that carnitine had anything to do with their season outcome, yet such advertising sells many bottles of carnitine.

Your body makes its own carnitine and distributes it to many of your body's cells. Primarily, it works to carry unoxidized fatty acids. These acids have a D form and an L form. Those initials just tell how the molecule rotates—to the right (dextro-, or D rotatory) or left (levo-rotatory, or L form.) Eating too much of the D form of carnitine in supplements can make you lose the L form. In this case, supplementation can be harmful.

It is difficult to become carnitine deficient through training. No good evidence suggests that taking carnitine in any of its forms does much that can be considered helpful, but we do not have enough evidence to reject it completely. Some studies show minor gains. For the small gains and big price, the average exerciser can gains as much and more through regular exercise.

Carnosine

Carnosine a compound made of amino acids. It is thought to have antioxidant properties. Some claims suggest that vegetarians might not get enough carnosine, as it is found only in meat. You manufacture carnosine in your own body. It is not an essential nutrient, meaning you don't need to eat it to have enough. Your body makes more antioxidants when you exercise.

Carbohydrate Injection

Korean speed skaters were reported to have been experimenting with glycogen injections directly into thigh muscle. For elite athletes, it is not known if it can be used or beneficial. The answer for regular exercisers is that it is completely unnecessary.

Fluid Retention

Fluid retention has been examined as an ergogenic aid. The theory is that muscle leverage favorably changes as the muscle swells with extra water. You can increase your total body water in several ways—carbohydrate loading increases the water your muscles can hold, eating salt retains more water, and anabolic steroids swell you with water, before they have a chance to exert any androgenic effect.

But should you count on fluid retention to help you in sports or exercise? Most people don't drink enough water, which is a common, and hidden, cause of fatigue. Getting enough water is a good idea and can make you feel better by itself. As far as dosing on extra water, the effect would be small, if any. Your body will usually regulate things so that any excess is quickly eliminated.

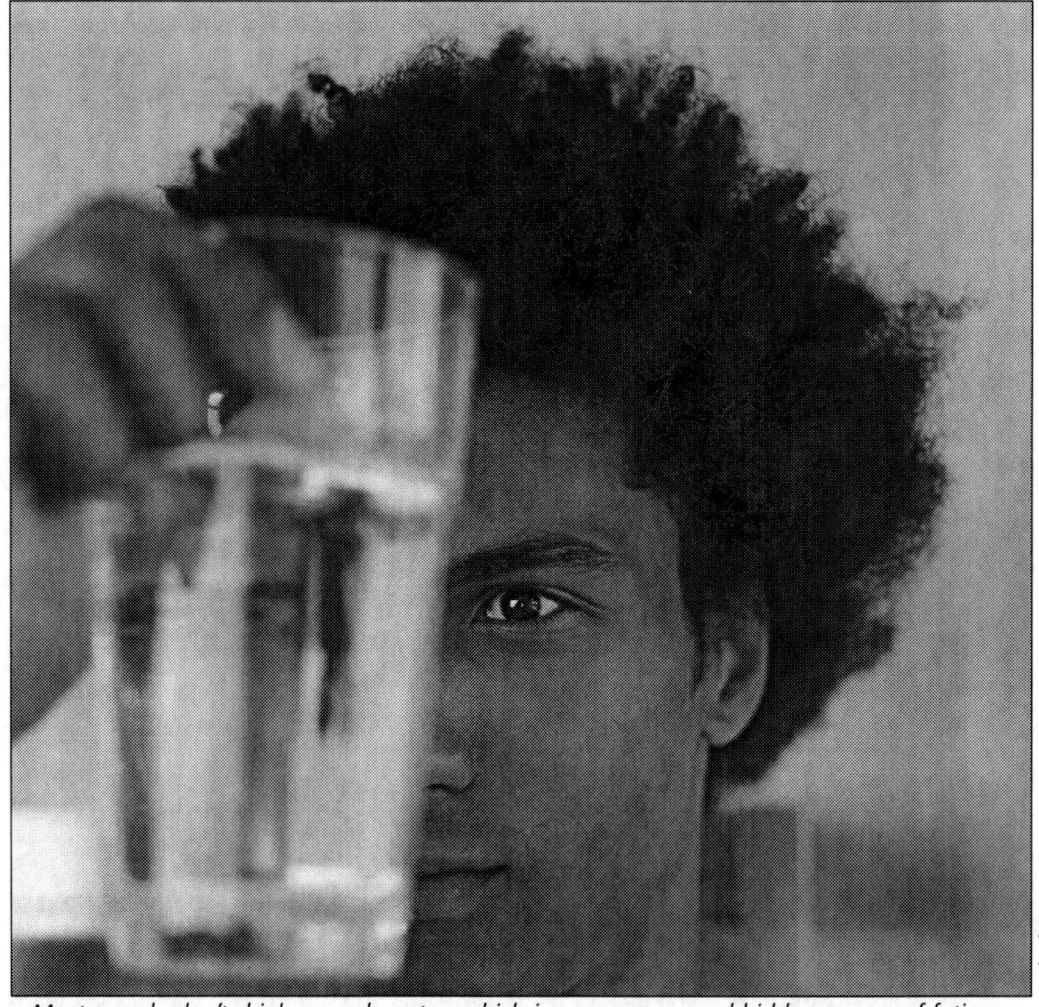

Most people don't drink enough water, which is a common, and hidden, cause of fatigue.

Water

For exercise, you need enough water to distribute to your skin for cooling and your muscles for working. Without enough to go around, you may overheat or not work at strong capacity. People overdo carrying water with them for minor exercise in air-conditioned gyms. If you are so dry that you cannot get through an hour of ordinary exercise without a bottle in your hand, you may have started out underhydrated.

Expensive bottled water is not always better or cleaner than tap water. Plastic bottles create a substantial problem of litter and waste in manufacture, transport, and disposal, harming the fitness of the environment. Chapter 10 provides ideas on making your own fitness water and drinks, and using filtered tap water in your own healthful, non-disposable containers.

Despite various fad-diet advice that extra large quantities of water must be consumed every day, or that large quantities of water will somehow remove substances, vaguely labeled "toxins," these claims have no solid support. Drinking enough good, clean water is important, healthy, and can help control appetite. Drink more water in the heat. Eating fruit and vegetables supplies water in healthy form. Drinking too much water will not make you healthier. Too much water, like many other things, is not good. Claims that you must drink eight glasses of water per day have little basis.

Avoid the Hype

Masses of products crowding store shelves claim to fix this and cure that. Product sales have risen to billions of dollars annually. Products seem dazzling, but much is hype and many produce unhealthful effects. More dollars follow on pills and products for problems that result, then more medicines when ill effects result in turn. Stop the cycle, and save time, money, and unhappiness. If it is not healthy, it is not health care.

What Will Give You an Advantage?

Regular good nutrition, good hydration, and regular exercise (not supplements) give true athletic advantage. What can you do?

- Eat a healthful breakfast. Include real raw fruit and nuts rather than toast and jam or processed cereal.
- Do not eat fast food or junk food.
- Know the difference between simple sugars and complex carbohydrates. Eat complex carbohydrates for the vitamins, nutrients, and energy-giving fuel you need for activity.

- Get enough protein early in the day. Don't have a coffee and Danish for breakfast and a salad for lunch. Get protein from vegetables and nuts, throughout the day. You'll sleep better without a high-protein dinner at night.
- Rest is a greatly ignored ergogenic aid. Get enough sleep, and enjoy your life.
- Exercise for fun and health.
- Drink water instead of commercial sport drinks or store-bought juice.
- Make your own juice with the pulp by putting your favorite fruit with clean water in a blender or mixer or get exercise by mashing it by hand.
- Make your own sport drinks instead of drinking sugar water in plastic bottles.
- Cut back (or out) on stimulants. Vicious cycles of dependence build. Stop unhealthy food, drink, and life habits that sap energy.
- Get outdoors in the sunshine (or the rain or snow) safely every day.
- Add up all the money you save on supplements. You will have enough to give to the poor and take a vacation.
- Be good to your mind and your body—a neglected personal-enhancing device.

CHAPTER 12
SPORT SUPPLEMENT BASICS

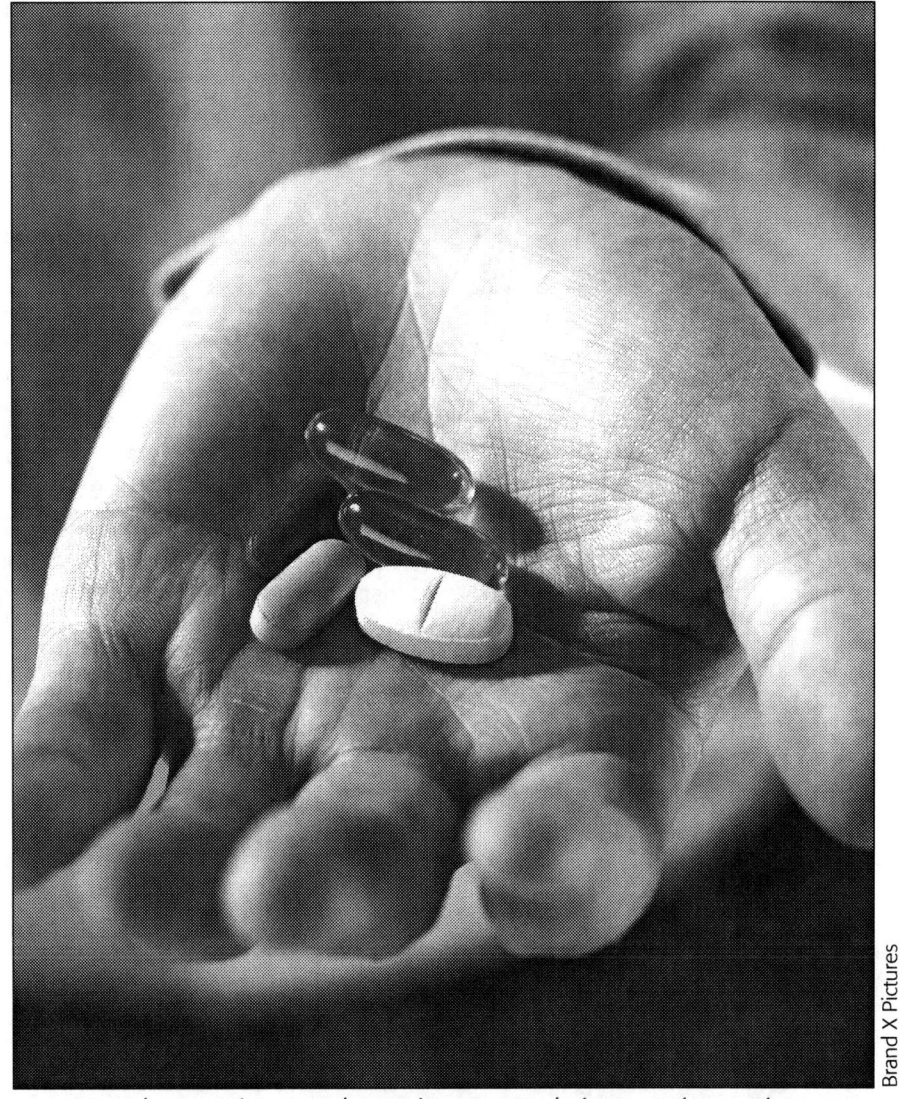

Supplementation can play an important role in correcting nutrient deficiencies in athletes who have poor diets and/or who fail to take into account the greater nutrient requirements of heavy training.

It is virtually impossible to go into a health food store and not see a wide variety of nutritional supplements available for purchase. Supplements are available in all sizes, brands, and mixtures, leaving consumers in a potential maze of confusion. In fact, it has been estimated that more than 600 dietary supplement manufacturers are located in the United States alone, producing more than 4,000 products totaling annual sales in excess of four to six billion dollars. Which of these supplements should athletes consume? This question is of major concern throughout athletics and may put athletes in a serious quandary. On one hand, athletes want to perform to their maximum potential, which requires optimizing the three major components of success: proper training, recovery, and nutrition. Certainly, the difference between a win and loss, or between first place and fifth place, will depend upon athletes' strength, muscular and cardiovascular endurance, body composition (i.e., the amount of body fat and muscle mass), power, skill and technique, speed, and agility—all of which are affected by dietary nutrient intake. On the other hand, athletes need to be concerned about critical elements such as the cost of supplements, potential side effects or negative health ramifications, ethics, and the potential for a failed drug test due to the intake of certain supplements.

In 1994, Congress passed the Dietary Supplement Health and Education Act (DSHEA). This document defines a supplement as "a product (other than tobacco) intended to supplement the diet that bears or contains one or more of the following dietary ingredients: a vitamin, a mineral, an herb or other botanical, an amino acid, a dietary substance for use by man to supplement the diet by increasing the total daily intake, or a concentrate, metabolite, constituent, extract, or combination of these ingredients." Although this document highlights the importance of supplements for improving health and reducing the risk factors for disease—as well as the importance of the supplement industry as an integral part of the economy—it also made it easier for supplement manufacturers to market their products. Prior to this document, federal legislation passed in 1993 limited the jurisdiction of the Food and Drug Administration (FDA) for regulating the quality, safety, and testing of nutrition supplements. The resulting situation—a combination of marketing ease and a lack of regulation—has contributed to the dramatic increase in sport supplement marketing and sales.

With the wealth of supplement information available, what do athletes need to know? Several key questions are addressed in this chapter that provide an overview of the supplementation process:

- How are supplements classified?
- Do athletes get their optimal nutrient requirements from diet alone?
- Can supplements provide additional benefits beyond what is provided by the diet?
- What is the physiological relevance of a supplement?
- Are supplement labels accurately represented?
- Does the cost of supplements outweigh the benefits?

- Should the age and the training experience of the athlete influence the decision to use nutrition supplements?
- Is supplementation popular among athletes?
- Does the supplement get to where it needs to be in the body?
- Does a dose-response pattern of improvement exist with supplementation?
- Should supplements be taken individually, or do they work better when taken in conjunction with other supplements?
- Can supplements be toxic when taken in doses far exceeding the recommended range?
- Does a placebo effect exist?
- What are responders and nonresponders?
- Is supplementation ethical?

General Classes of Supplements

Supplements are classified based on their functions in the human body:

- *Macronutrients* are those nutrients required in large amounts from a person's diet and include proteins, carbohydrates, fats, and water, which make up approximately 60 to 70 percent of a person's body weight. Proteins are made up of building blocks called amino acids, which have functions both individually and collectively. Some amino acid–related compounds also play key roles in cellular processes, and some show potential ergogenic benefits.
- *Micronutrients* are needed in much smaller amounts in the human diet, but, nevertheless, perform life-sustaining functions in the body. Micronutrients include vitamins and minerals.
- *Prohormones*—which are, in fact, hormones—are precursor molecules involved ultimately in the biosynthesis of testosterone.
- *Cellular metabolism supplements* perform multiple functions in skeletal muscle, such as acid-base buffering, energy production, material transport, and volumizing (i.e., increasing the solute concentration such as creatine phosphate within the cells). These supplements may also be included within other multipurpose supplements.
- *Thermogenic supplements* increase metabolism. By increasing the metabolism, an individual can achieve body-fat reductions and possibly affect acute performance, depending on the compound in question (e.g., some thermogenic molecules may impact strength, endurance, and mental focus during exercise).
- *Antioxidants* help control the damaging effects of free radicals on cells in the body. A number of nutrients function as antioxidants, and these act collectively to reduce tissue damage and promote health.

Other supplements have been classified in more general terms. For example, weight-gain, weight-loss, and recovery supplements typically contain multiple nutrients that perform similar functions. *Weight-gain powders and drinks* typically contain high-calorie mixtures of macronutrients, as well as fortification with vitamins and minerals. *Weight-loss supplements* may contain thermogenic compounds, which are micronutrients involved in fat-burning or energy-producing reactions, and appetite suppressants, as well as other cofactors and micronutrients. Multipurpose supplements contain combinations of compounds that may enhance more than one aspect of performance. For example, *recovery supplements* may include large concentrations of carbohydrates, proteins, and some micronutrients, but may also include creatine, ß-hydroxy-ß-methylbutyrate (HMB), antioxidants, glutamine, and other compounds that improve physical function by different means. In addition, pharmacological agents (which require a prescription or may be banned by sport-governing bodies) are also common.

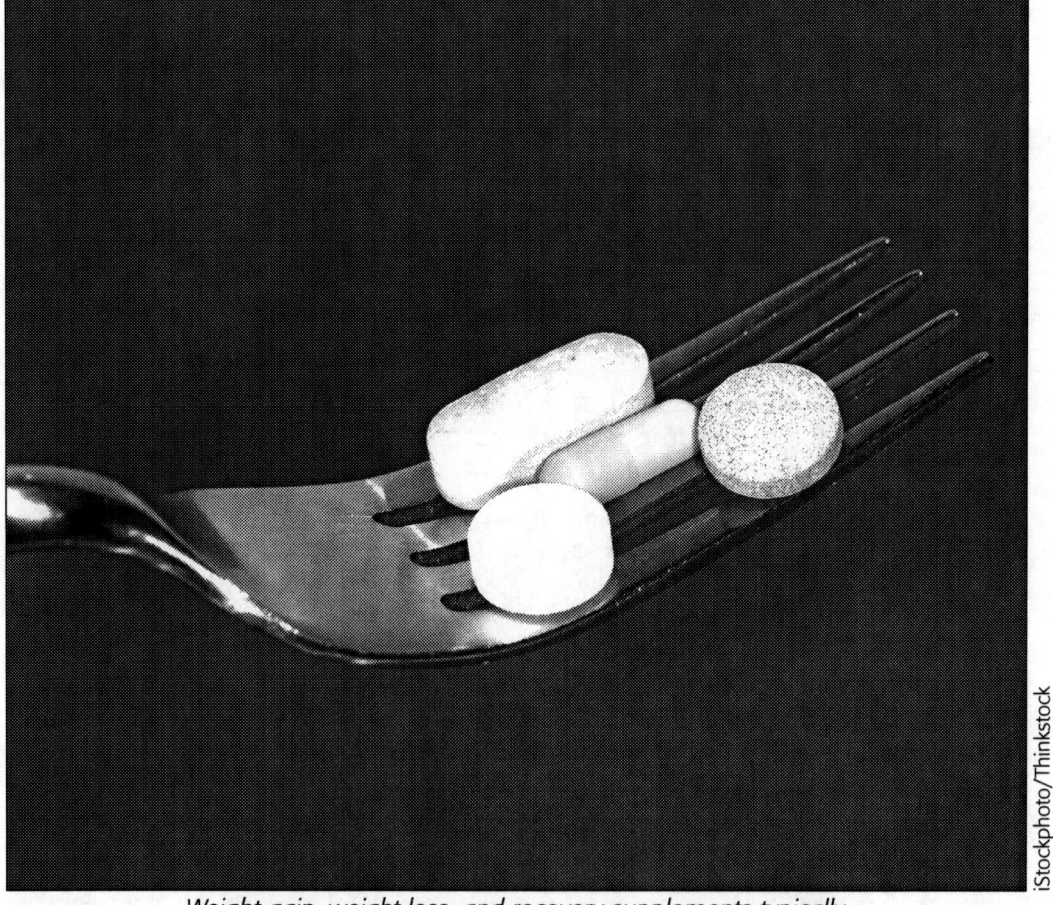

Weight-gain, weight-loss, and recovery supplements typically contain multiple nutrients that perform similar functions.

Nutrient Deficiency

A deficiency indicates a lack of, or a suboptimal intake of, one or more nutrients that are essential to optimal bodily function. Supplementation can play an important role in correcting nutrient deficiencies in athletes who have poor diets and/or who fail to take into account the greater nutrient requirements of heavy training. Some athletes may be deficient in certain macro- or micronutrients, and supplementation can help correct these deficiencies. With the rigors of off- and in-season training, practice, and competition, the nutrient needs of an athlete are far greater than those of a non-athlete. If these needs are not met, the athlete may be at a disadvantage.

It is important to note that nutrients work in synergy. In other words, for one nutrient to function properly, balance must be attained among other nutrients that perform similar functions or are involved in the same reaction. For example, vitamins and minerals serve as cofactors in bodily reactions. Because multiple vitamins or minerals are involved in certain reactions, a deficiency in only one can limit the process or slow down the reactions. A common example is Vitamin E and selenium, as these micronutrients work in synergy as antioxidants. Therefore, supplements that correct deficiencies can enhance performance, but they are not truly ergogenic because they would provide no further benefit if dietary intake was adequate.

To achieve adequate dietary intake of all essential nutrients, athletes must increase the amount of food and beverages they consume. This task may be difficult, especially during the midst of a heavy training, practice, and competition schedule. Additional time constraints from school and/or work may also exist, thereby causing the athlete some degree of difficulty in maintaining a consistent meal plan. Training, practice, and competition—especially in hot, humid weather—have the additional antagonizing effect of reducing the athlete's appetite. When taking all of these variables into consideration, the difficulty facing an athlete when trying to consume sufficient macro- and micronutrients solely from the diet becomes more evident. This scenario provides an example of when supplementation gives an athlete a competitive edge.

The ability to consume nutrients from non-food sources becomes important for preventing a deficiency. Sport supplements provide another practical advantage for athletes. Because many sport supplements are available in liquid or powder form (where the powder is mixed into a liquid drink) or as health bars, they provide essential nutrients rapidly and with great flexibility of consumption (i.e., they can easily be transported or consumed any time of day, including those times when the athlete is in class, at work, etc., and may have limited access to food). In addition, sport supplement drinks can quench thirst and rehydrate athletes during training, practice, and competition. They are more easily digestible than a meal, which gives the athlete quicker access to nutrients. Therefore, sport supplements provide several advantages to athletes in the quest to minimize the risk of nutritional deficiency.

Ergogenic Supplements

The term "ergogenic" refers to performance or work enhancement. It originates from the Greek *ergon* (meaning "work") and *gennan* (meaning "to produce"). In supplement terms, a chemical compound that enhances performance beyond that of normal dietary intake of that compound is considered ergogenic. By this definition, an ergogenic supplement should enhance some facet of performance when no nutrient deficiency is observed. Ergogenic supplements may:

- Increase muscle strength and power
- Increase muscle size
- Increase muscular endurance and reduce fatigue
- Enhance immune-system function and recovery between workouts
- Increase energy availability and reduce body fat
- Improve specific parameters of sport performance

Many supplement labels claim that product to be ergogenic. Manufacturers of nutrition supplements have as their sole purpose the marketing and selling of their products. Therefore, exaggerated claims are not uncommon. Athletes must be aware of unsubstantiated claims that may tempt them to purchase a supplement. Additional scientific studies are needed to properly investigate the ergogenic potential of supplement use. Sport scientists carefully design studies by doing the following:

- Using a placebo (i.e., a "fake" supplement) as a control in such as way that neither the investigator nor the athlete knows what is being taken (to avoid bias)
- Administering precise doses of the supplement to the athletes
- Including a sufficient number of athletes to get strong statistical power
- Minimizing any confounding effects from extraneous factors that are not part of the study
- Precisely measuring performance and physiological variables that the supplement may affect
- Implementing proper training protocols to accurately reveal the supplement's utility

Some supplements display scientific references on the label to substantiate use of that product. While this practice can be helpful, some deception can take place, as research findings are often taken out of context.

In terms of ergogenicity, many supplements get a failing grade by rigorous scientific standards. Many supplements have failed to enhance performance when consumed at the manufacturer's recommended dosages. However, it is quite common to see athletes consume nutrition supplements at doses that far exceed the recommended range. Anecdotally, testimonials in several magazine articles, advertisements, and interviews with well-known athletes have suggested some of these supplements to be ergogenic when taken at supraphysiological doses. However, few scientific studies have examined supplement doses in that high range, so it is unclear if the statements have any merit. Using consistency as a standard, only a few supplements have repeatedly proven to be advantageous.

Physiological Relevance of Supplement Use

The key questions to ask when appraising potential supplements for use are: What is the supplement's physiological relevance, and what is the supplement supposed to do? The answers to these questions may require some background knowledge of physiology. The supplement in question must have some involvement in the processes affecting acute and chronic performance and training adaptations. If the supplement appears to have no benefit on the surface, then that supplement is likely not worthy of use physiologically or economically.

Supplement Use Among Athletes

Sport supplement use in athletes has increased in popularity over the years. Historically, athletic departments were allowed to distribute supplements to student-athletes. However, that practice is no longer tolerated, as controversies involving some supplements (e.g., creatine, prohormones, and ephedra) have led to imposed limitations on supplement distribution by the athletic department. Nevertheless, student-athletes still have unlimited access to sport supplements provided they are purchased outside of the school setting. One study by Burns et al (2004) showed that out of eight NCAA I universities, 80 percent of the 228 athletes surveyed reported using one supplement and 58 percent reported using at least two sport supplements as part of their training. Most studies have shown that, on average, more than 50 percent of athletes consume nutrition supplements, and the higher the level of competition, the greater the prevalence of supplement use (i.e., elite athletes are the most frequent consumers). Among the supplements consumed, vitamin/minerals, calorie-replacement drinks, proteins/amino acids, and creatine are the most popular.

Although elite athletes may be the predominant supplement consumers, a trickle-down effect exists, and young athletes are supplementing more now than ever before. High school and middle school student-athletes are becoming aware of the popularity of sport supplements through friends, magazines, and the media (e.g., reports of famous athletes using supplements). Great pressure to win from coaches, parents, and friends, coupled with the fact that some athletes are now turning professional out of high school, may cause young athletes to view supplement use as a means to achieving greater success. In fact, a 2001 study by Metzl et al looked at creatine use in sixth through twelfth grades and found that approximately 6 percent of students had taken creatine. The highest rate was observed in twelfth graders (44 percent), and gymnastics, hockey, wrestling, football, lacrosse, and weight training were the sports and activities that saw the highest incidence of creatine use. When the scientists investigated potential reasons for creatine use among these populations, the most common responses were enhanced performance, appearance, speed, and endurance.

Other popular supplements among high school athletes are multivitamins and minerals, amino acid and protein, weight gainers, HMB, sport drinks, and prohormones (although prohormones have been banned from over-the-counter sales). A 2004 study by Bartee et al revealed the following trends among 1,737 ninth through twelfth graders surveyed:

- Boys had an 87 percent greater chance of using supplements than girls.
- Twelfth graders were 64 percent more likely to supplement than ninth graders.
- Students who participated in two or more sports were most likely to supplement.
- Athletes with a favorable outlook on supplement use had a 13 times greater likelihood of consuming supplements.
- Athletes with supportive parents or guardians were more likely to use supplements.

Interestingly, a study by Massad et al (1995) showed that supplement use declined when high school athletes were educated properly about supplements.

Sources of Supplement Knowledge Among Athletes

Where athletes get their information on sport supplements is very important. Due to the mass marketing of supplements and exaggerated claims on labels and in advertisements, it is very easy for athletes to be fed misinformation. Virtually every supplement advertisement claims some ergogenic element that enhances performance, which leaves the athlete in a tempting situation. Athletes should refer to credible sources on sport supplements. In Division I athletics, athletic trainers and strength and conditioning coaches are often sought out for supplement information. However, other reports show that friends, teammates, and magazines are often prime sources of supplement information, which means that the chances of athletes receiving misinformation are very likely. It is essential for athletes to properly educate themselves.

Athletes' Age and Level of Training

At what age should athletes begin taking nutrition supplements? The answer to this question is not simple, as many young athletes become fascinated with the supplement industry and some experiment with supplements at an early age, especially since some of their professional athlete role models are spokespersons for various supplements. Many young athletes feel compelled to start supplementing early to get ahead of the competition. Athletes turning pro out of high school do very little to curtail this phenomenon. The basic premise is that if it helps, then the young athlete will try it. But, should this trend be the norm or the exception?

The key element is the level of maturity and training experience of the young athlete. Teenagers' bodies are still in the developmental stage. Growth spurts take place at periodic phases and hormonal changes are evident, meaning that the possibility of training adaptations is still very large and normal dietary intake supplies adequate amounts of nutrients to sustain training at this level. Perhaps a multivitamin or some additional carbohydrates and protein may be useful at this stage, but other supplements do not appear necessary in most cases. Historically, supplement use has been most effective when used to overcome training plateaus. That is, many individuals (especially resistance-trained athletes such as strength competitors, bodybuilders, Olympic weight lifters, and power lifters) establish a firm training base during the first few years of training and later use supplements when progression becomes more difficult. With this model in mind, it makes sense for young athletes to train smart and eat right initially, develop a firm conditioning base, and then supplement in later years (i.e., late teens to early twenties). Using this technique, supplements may be used in a more efficient manner to surpass plateaus when gains become somewhat more difficult to obtain.

A prime example of establishing a training base before supplementing is evident in a common criticism of several sport supplement studies. Some research studies have been criticized for using previously untrained individuals as subjects due to the high learning curve associated with the initial training phase. It is a fact that adaptations of the nervous system predominate early in training, and untrained subjects respond favorably regardless of the training program. Testing a supplement or even a training program at this point is extremely difficult because any potential differentiating effects may be overshadowed by the learning curve. For example, some creatine supplementation studies have shown no ergogenic benefits in untrained subjects (although some studies have shown benefits). But why use a known ergogenic at a time when gains should be prevalent anyway? These studies lack a practical application, but an analogy can be made to young athletes. As long as gains are being made through training alone, sport supplements may not be necessary until the rate of progression has slowed significantly.

An exception to this model may be caused by the level of competition encountered by the athlete. Young, elite athletes competing in sports in which peak performance and success may be attained at a young age (e.g., gymnastics) may benefit from the use of some supplements. Competing at that elite level may supersede typical supplementation guidelines.

Bioavailability: Does the Supplement Get to Where It Needs to Be?

Bioavailability refers to how much of a consumed supplement actually reaches the target site. The supplement needs to end up in its proper location for the desired effects to occur. Bioavailability is determined by the nature and formulation of the supplement. For example, L-carnitine has been used as a "fat burner" because of its role as a transporter of fatty acids in the muscle's mitochondria (i.e., the site of aerobic energy metabolism within the cell). Although supplementation studies have shown a higher level of L-carnitine in the blood, no elevation in L-carnitine concentration within the muscle has been documented. These results show that supplemental L-carnitine does not reach the target area, which casts doubt on the effectiveness of its use in this context. In fact, some studies have shown no effect on body composition with L-carnitine supplementation.

Supplement Patterns

The pattern of supplementation refers to the method by which the supplement is taken. In other words, is it more effective to take a constant dose of a supplement regularly over a long period of time or to "cycle" a supplement based on the training phase? The answer depends on the supplement in question. Supplements used to correct a deficiency are most often taken at consistent doses over a period of time. Supplementing with 400 international units (IU) of Vitamin E per day over the course of a year is a common example. Taking more than the needed amount provides no further benefit. Therefore, a constant dose is sufficient to maintain optimal levels of intake.

Considering that the majority of benefits that occur with "ergogenic" supplements take place during the initial phase of supplementation, some authorities have suggested that cycling supplements may be more effective for getting a more substantial, long-term effect. Cycling refers to a pattern of use in which the athlete takes the supplement for a period of time (usually 6 to 12 weeks), and then reduces the dose over time until use of the supplement is terminated. After a period of training without the supplement, the athlete will then initiate another cycle further into the training period. The rationale behind cycling is to increase performance during supplementation, maintain as much of the performance gain as possible without supplement use (i.e., a residual effect), and begin a new supplementation cycle at a higher training base than the previous cycle. A supplement with which cycling may be useful is creatine.

Label Accuracy

An accurately labeled supplement is important to the athlete. Stated simply, the supplement should be composed of what is stated on the label. Although the United States Food and Drug Administration set standards for the testing, promotion, and advertising of prescription drugs, sport supplements are less tightly controlled. The impact of a mislabeled supplement on the athlete could be as simple as a supplement that is less effective, or it could mean the possibility of a failed drug test if the supplement is contaminated with a banned substance such as a prohormone or anabolic steroid.

Dose Response and Toxicity

A dose-response relationship indicates how much of an effect is obtained from the supplement at various levels of consumption. For most supplements that correct a deficiency in athletes, the amount of supplement taken may be more than the recommended daily allowance (RDA). Therefore, any more will be of no additional benefit. Activity level, as well as other circumstances, increases the nutrient requirements. Taking more than what is necessary provides no further advantage to an athlete. For some ergogenic supplements that are pharmaceutical in nature, a more sufficient response may be present with gradually increasing doses. Nevertheless, a common—and erroneous—thought is that if X amount of a supplement works, then increasing the dose substantially to Y will have a greater effect. The truth is that athletes taking supraphysiological doses of supplements over an extended period of time run the risk of toxicity, a negative health manifestation due to consumption of too large a dose of supplements.

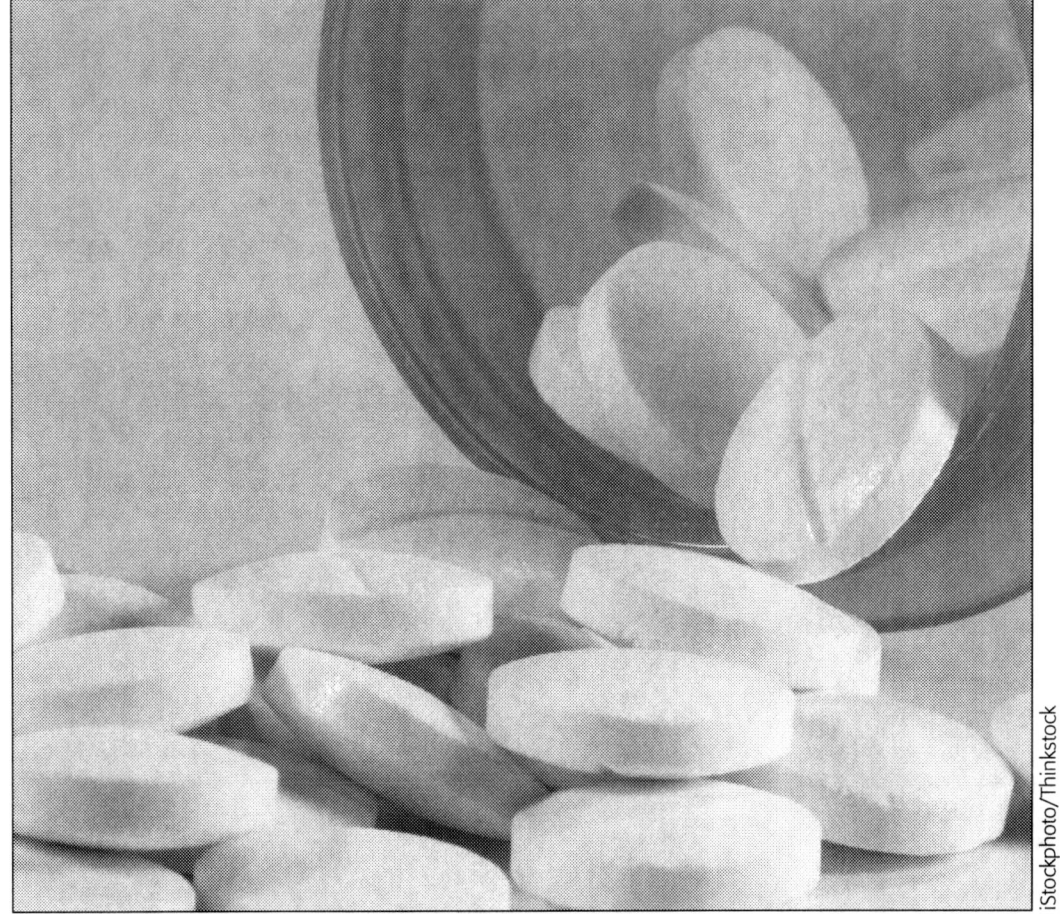

A common—and erroneous—thought is that if X amount of a supplement works, then increasing the dose substantially to Y will have a greater effect.

The Placebo Effect

A psychological component exists with supplementation. In some instances, the athlete thinks the supplement will enhance performance and he subsequently trains harder. Improvement in performance may occur, but this improvement is most likely due to the athlete's enhanced training initiative and not to the supplement itself. The improvement occurs as a result of what is called the placebo effect. A placebo is a fake (in the sense that it has no physiological value) pill or powder given to subjects or patients in studies as a control to investigate the effects of another drug or supplement. Many times, an athlete's improved performance has been falsely attributed to a particular supplement when, in fact, the athlete was training more intensely under the assumption that the supplement was working. The placebo effect is yet another reason why it is important to base decisions on scientifically controlled studies rather than anecdotal information.

Responders vs. Nonresponders

Many studies that have shown the ergogenic properties of supplements do not have 100 percent of the subjects showing the same rate of improvement. In some cases, some subjects do not improve at all. A responder is an athlete who achieves a high level of performance enhancement from supplementation. A nonresponder, therefore, is someone who receives very little, if any, benefit. Scientists have tried to identify reasons why some individuals have no response when the majority of subjects/athletes in a study experience improvements. Although the reasons are not clear, there is plenty of evidence that genetic factors play a role in these individual physiological differences (e.g., muscle-fiber composition).

CHAPTER 13
GETTING TO THE RIGHT WEIGHT
AND BODY COMPOSITION FOR ATHLETIC SUCCESS

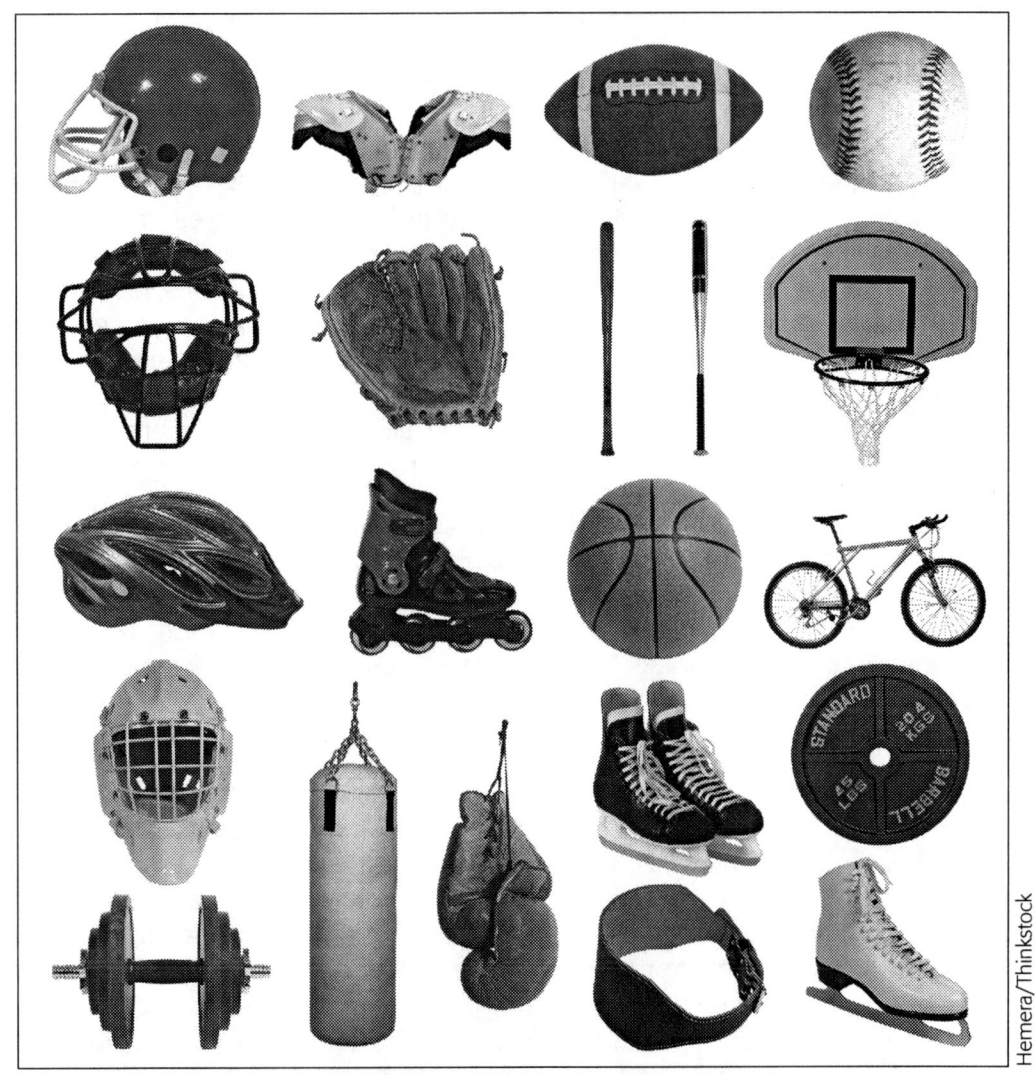

The principles behind controlling body weight and maintaining good health are essentially the same. The health of the athlete is as important as weight loss or weight gain for athletic success.

The most advantageous body weight (or body composition) for athletes has been a significant issue for coaches, athletes, parents, school administrators, family members, friends, and a wide spectrum of health care providers for many decades. Since the identification and recognition of "weight classes" in sports such as wrestling, boxing, judo, and weightlifting, athletes have been obsessively reducing body weight to the lowest possible level while potentially compromising strength, endurance, and agility. "Cutting weight" has become an athletic national pastime that has simultaneously intrigued and horrified coaches, athletes, physicians, athletic trainers, exercise physiologists, and nutritionists. In some sports, even those with no identifiable weight classes for athletes (such as gymnasts, ice skaters, and jockeys), the problem is no different. A third group of athletes includes those who are compulsive about weight loss because their bodies are exposed by the required uniforms of the sport.

However, advantages do exist in some sports for reducing body weight (especially if it is in the form of body fat). For example, athletes who compete in sports that require jumping or running (e.g., gymnastics, pole vault, high jump, sprinting) are often at an advantage at lower body weights, but the advantages are only up to a point and performance often decreases after some baseline level is surpassed. If a little bit is good, it does not mean going further in reduction of body fat percentage is better. These athletes do very well with a reduced body-fat percentage and an increased lean body mass, which is composed mostly of muscle. These same athletes would not perform as well if they were to add body weight in the form of fat weight (a simple law of physics). Therefore, these athletes would do well to reduce body weight to the lowest percentage of body fat possible, while still maintaining the much-needed strength, endurance, and agility to perform at their very best.

The problem that exists among this group of athletes is the determination of the optimal body weight at which they will excel. For many athletes, only trial and error will answer that question—something that most athletes are not willing to do. Therefore, the weight-reduction routines continue because the athlete (and the coach) do not know any better and are not willing (understandably) to experiment with different body weights. The succession of weight loss and weight gain continues as the athlete cycles into and out of a season.

Some athletes actually strive to gain weight before and during a competitive season. Interior linemen on a football team are an example of a group of athletes who typically have difficulty maintaining their body weights. Interior football linemen are, by their very nature, large human beings. Their position on a football team requires them to move aside other players who are just as large. The laws of physics suggest that it is easier for the larger player to move the smaller player out of the way (technique and skill aside). The issue facing these types of players is gaining weight and maintaining that weight over the course of the football season. It is not unlikely that a football player will expend more than 6,000 calories on any given day. To replace those calories, the right kinds of foods must be introduced into the diet. The replacement calories should have a purpose and not just be any kind of food the athlete desires.

The principles behind controlling body weight and maintaining good health are essentially the same. The health of the athlete is as important as weight loss or weight gain for athletic success. This chapter, then, addresses these issues as though they were the same. While the prevalence of eating disorders in the athletic population is well documented, this book only describes these important psychological and medical conditions. The athlete should refer to a medical or behavioral health professional if an eating disorder is suspected. Instead, this book discusses the proper ways to lose weight, maintain weight, or gain weight in athletic populations. Athletes who are concerned about anorexia nervosa, bulimia nervosa, and other eating disorders should consult with their physicians. Likewise, athletes who are concerned about obesity should consult with a medical team consisting of a medical doctor, a behavior therapist, and a registered dietitian, who can help treat the condition.

Energy Balance

All sports have some degree of physical resistance associated with them. For example, ice skaters have to overcome the resistance of the skate blade and the ice, cyclists have to overcome air resistance and forces created from the pedal to the tire and from the tire to the ground, powerlifters have to overcome the resistance of the weights, and divers and gymnasts experience resistance on the diving board and on each apparatus, respectively. Sport performance is related to athletes' ability to overcome the imposed resistance, and their ability to sustain high levels of power output by doing so. Athletes typically confuse the ability to overcome this imposed resistance with the ability to carry a lot of muscle and a relatively little amount of fat. It is true that fat mass, in most sports, does little to contribute to high levels of performance. However, the strategy that many athletes have used is to reduce fat mass and increase muscle mass through a calorie-restricted diet (dramatically lowering total energy intake), which is counterproductive because it restricts the intake of energy that is needed to sustain the energy required for the activity. Overcoming resistance and sustaining power are related to performance, but are perceived by many athletes to be conflicting. This misunderstanding often causes the athlete to reduce caloric intake when energy demand is highest.

The answer to this question may lie in the ability of athletes to balance their energy intake with their energy demands throughout the entire day (and not at the traditional three meals each day). Energy balance has been the subject of much study. Most athletes want to simultaneously increase muscle mass while reducing fat mass. The dilemma has been to find a dietary program that coincides with the practice schedule, game or competition schedule, and the daily energy needs of the athlete that also emphasizes an increase in lean body mass (muscle) and a reduction in fat mass. A number of very good scientific studies have suggested that the answer may be in consuming small but frequent meals to stay in better energy balance throughout the day, regardless of the practice or competition schedule.

Traditionally, energy balance has been assessed over a 24-hour period. Nutritionists would calculate the total number of calories consumed and the total number of calories expended. If the athlete consumed 3,200 calories during the day and "burned" 3,200 calories during the same day, he was thought to be in an "energy balance" (same number of calories in as out). A better way to look at energy balance is to see what happens *during* the day and to discover how the athlete was able to achieve a state of energy balance.

An athlete could spend a majority of the day in an energy deficit (burning more calories than consumed at any specific period of time). Eating a large meal at the end of the day can satisfy the energy needs of the whole day as measured using the traditional methods of calculating energy balance. The athlete is back in an energy balance, but only at the end of the day. This kind of caloric payback at the end of the day may have serious implications for the athlete and his training program. When energy stores are called upon during a practice session or during a competition, when the athlete is in an energy deficit, the athlete must revert back to energy in the form of fats or even proteins, which are not the most efficient ways to secure energy because of the depletion of stored carbohydrates, which are the preferred energy source stored in the muscles.

Athletes who wait until the end of the day to replenish energy stores seem to have different competition or practice outcomes than those who are in an energy-balanced state throughout the day. An athlete has several advantages when eating smaller and more-frequent meals. For example, the resting metabolic rate dictates the number of calories expended without activity-related energy expenditure. Frequently eating small meals helps the metabolic rate stay the same throughout the day. It does not fluctuate as it does on the traditional three-meals-a-day plan. The athlete has enough energy to sustain his practice or competition schedule without mobilizing fats or proteins as the energy source. At the same time, numerous scientific studies have shown that a more frequent meal plan actually leads to a lower body fat, lower body weight, better maintenance of muscle mass, and improved physical performance.

Many coaches have recognized the physical and cognitive difficulties athletes typically have toward the end of long practices. In addition, American culture seems to dictate that people traditionally delay eating a large meal until the end of the day. This practice leads to severe energy deficits *during* the day, especially on those days when athletes train hardest and need the energy the most. Studies have consistently shown that numerous problems, including traumatic injury, are created when an athlete is in an energy deficit. Many of these problems are the opposite of the advantages found when an athlete consumes small but frequent meals.

As a result of eating a large meal, carbohydrates are absorbed from the small intestine into the liver. If a biological need exists to replenish muscle glucose (stored as glycogen), some of the glucose from the meal is transported to the muscle, where it is converted into stored glycogen, ready to be used the next time the athlete needs it.

The storage of glucose, however, is limited. Once glycogen stores have been maximized, no more need exists for the glucose circulating in the blood. As a response to this now excessive amount of glucose in the blood, the pancreas receives a message to reduce the blood glucose. The pancreas secretes insulin, which not only helps with the introduction of glucose into cells, but also drives down the glucose levels in the blood. Any additional absorbed glucose from the meal is converted to the storage form of excess glucose—fat.

After the meal, and once glycogen stores are at their maximal levels and the excess glucose has been converted to fat, the body starts to use glycogen while performing activities of daily living. If the athlete was to practice or compete several hours after a meal, he may not have sufficient stores of glycogen to perform at a high level. He would simply run out of available fuel. A more indirect consequence of eating large meals and the consistent cycling of eating and fasting is a reduction in the metabolic rate, which then corresponds to problems with maintaining lean muscle mass and a predisposition to injury.

Optimal Weight and Body Composition

A simple relationship exists between weight gain or weight loss and caloric intake. If an athlete eats more calories than he expends (or "burns"), he will eventually store the excess amount of calories as body fat and his weight will increase. When the athlete eats fewer calories than he expends, he will lose weight. If the athlete consumes the same number of calories as he expends, body weight will stay the same.

An athlete who is on a calorie-restricted diet and eats fewer calories than he will use during the day will call upon some existing body tissues for the needed energy (typically in the form of stored fat). As a result, body weight will decrease. At the point at which the amount of fat available for fuel is decreased and is no longer available as a source of energy, the body then turns to the next available source, which is protein. The consistent reliance on protein as the energy source causes the lean mass (muscles) to actually *decrease* the rate at which calories are burned (called the "metabolic rate"). The result of a chronically lowered metabolic rate is usually a *higher* body-fat level, because the body is less able to burn the calories consumed, resulting in more fat storage. Staying in an energy balance (or only deviating from it slightly) is an important strategy for maintaining body weight and body composition.

Athlete Weight-Loss Programs

For many generations of athletes, weight loss has led to significant acute and chronic medical conditions that have, in the worst cases, caused traumatic injury, and have commonly led to a decline in performance. In either case, the athlete can suffer a career-ending injury or realize a decline in strength that leads to a poor performance. Some of the same weight-loss practices of many years ago are still practiced today.

Numerous wrestlers today, for example, will still dehydrate or starve days before a match in order to "make weight."

The recommended method for athletes to lose weight is through balancing the caloric intake and output in favor of the output (refer to Figure 13-3). Athletes and their coaches preparing for a competitive season should determine the optimal weight for the athlete and then plan a weight-reduction program to meet those goals. It is understood that a 1- to 2-pound weight loss per week will lead to preserving lean body mass (muscle) while using stored fat as the source of energy during the dieting period. A greater weight loss may lead to a reduction in muscle mass because, during those periods of dieting, the body may call upon protein stores (i.e., muscle) to provide needed energy.

A caloric-output balance of approximately 3,500 calories in a week—which equates to a 500-calorie deficit each day—will yield a weight loss of one pound (0.45 kilograms). Dieting alone can often yield this kind of result very comfortably. In only two months of preseason training, with no additional caloric expenditure, an athlete can lose 10 pounds (4.5 kilograms) in 10 weeks. However, if the weight-loss goal was 20 pounds (9.1 kilograms) in that same time period, the weekly average goal would have to be 2 pounds (0.9 kilograms), which would require 1,000 calories expended over the amount consumed each day.

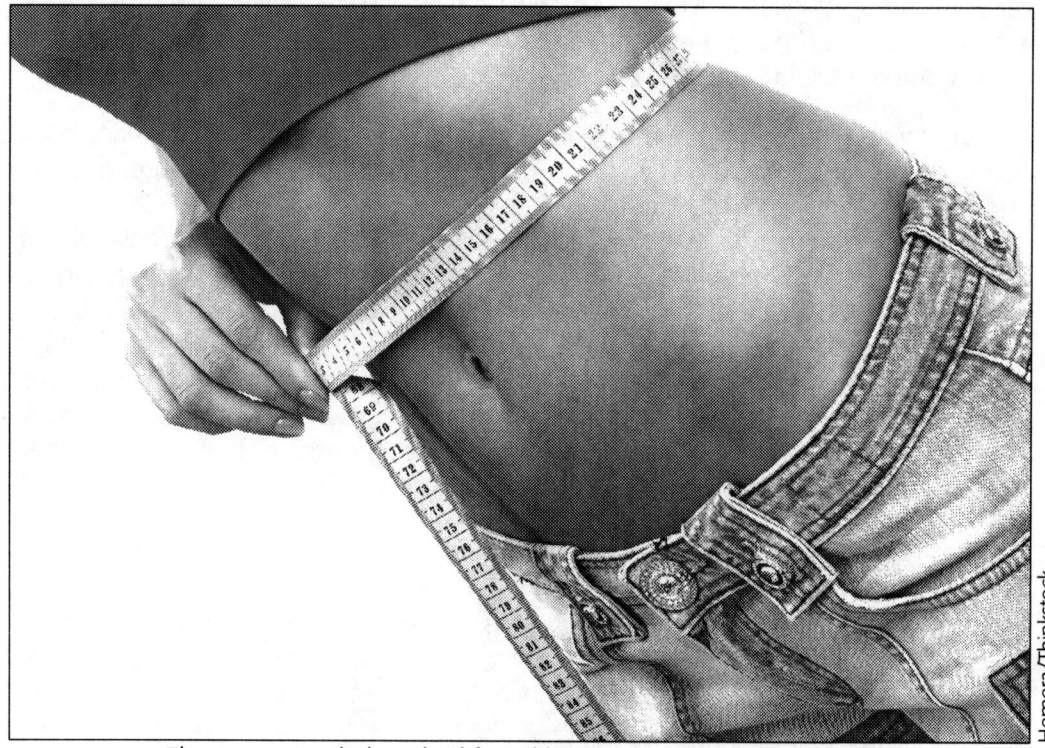

The recommended method for athletes to lose weight is through balancing the caloric intake and output in favor of the output.

Given that the average caloric intake of an athlete may be 3,000 calories, restricting the caloric intake to this degree would allow the athlete to consume only 2,000 calories (reducing his caloric intake by one third). This kind of caloric restriction would then place the athlete in danger of using some of the valuable protein stores (i.e., muscles) as an energy source. The better approach to the two-pounds-a-week (0.9 kilograms) weight-loss program would be to follow the same 500-calorie restriction in the previous example and then add a daily exercise program that would expend an additional 500 calories. The result would be the same 1,000-calorie deficit. In 10 weeks, the weight loss would be 20 pounds (9.1 kilograms). This approach is not only safer, but will preserve the athlete's strength and endurance.

Some athletes in weight-restricted sports may be pushing the upper limits of a weight class prior to each competition, particularly over the course of a season in which the athlete begins to gain lean mass just from the process of growth and maturation. Difficult decisions must be made to either allow the athlete to move up a weight class or to give up his spot on the team. Neither of these two solutions is typically satisfactory to the athlete. The most common solution is to sustain the acute weight-loss pattern over the course of the remaining competition season. This pattern is neither safe nor medically advised. A better solution is for a coach to monitor the athlete's weight from preseason through the season and to make sure no more than a 1-pound (0.45 kilogram) daily weight swing occurs.

Athletes will often have a competition on a Saturday (after a few days of dehydration and starvation), and then gorge themselves on food and drink Saturday night and all day on Sunday. It is not inconceivable that an athlete could gain between three and five pounds in just a day-and-a-half. Athletes who routinely practice this kind of acute weight gain will then have to lose that amount of weight (and more) to "make weight" the following weekend. This vicious cycling of weight loss and weight gain can last for several months—a practice that is hardly beneficial to the athlete, and may actually cause a decrement in performance.

A better practice for these athletes is to maintain the same weight throughout the week prior to competition. Athletes should not cycle through periods of feast and famine. They should be monitored for consistent body weight. Once an athlete reaches a certain body weight (not taking into consideration the effects of maturation and growth), it is easier to maintain that weight than to gain weight post-competition and then have to lose the weight during the following practice sessions. A consistent body weight (assisted by eating frequent meals) held throughout the competition season is healthier and leads to the maintaining of strength and endurance for a longer period of time.

Athlete Weight-Gain Programs

Many athletes are more interested in weight gain than weight loss. In fact, more athletes want to gain weight than lose weight during the preseason and competitive season. The problem, however, is excess weight gained in the form of body fat and not muscle. For many athletes, proper weight gain will be accomplished by increasing lean body mass. Strength training will often increase muscle mass, even when the athlete is in a minor caloric deficit. The energy in the case of an athlete who strength trains will come first from carbohydrate stores (which are easily replaced), followed by stored fat, as long as the caloric restriction is temporary.

Athletes who compete in power-type sports often wish to increase muscle mass and typically do so by adding strength training to their practice schedules. In addition to the strength training, it is advisable to add a small amount of protein to the diet. No reason exists to take a protein supplement, however. With the increase in caloric consumption by these athletes to maintain energy balance (so they do not lose weight), an increase typically takes place in the amount of protein in the diet, which is usually at a sufficient level to take care of rebuilding muscle tissues. It is recommended that athletes increase their protein consumption from 0.8 grams per kilogram of body weight to 1.6 (doubling the amount of protein in the diet). Most sport nutritionists believe that athletes increase the protein intake without any changes in the diet, by simply increasing caloric consumption. The major issue created by increasing the protein consumption in the diet is the same as that created when increasing carbohydrates. The excess protein (i.e., protein not used for rebuilding muscle tissue) is converted to fat—the same kind of fat created by excess consumption of carbohydrates.

In a positive energy balance, excess calories are converted to stored fat. Excess protein intake in the form of food or a dietary supplement is not excreted as is typically thought. The increase in urine output of protein after a strength-training workout can be traced to the degradation of muscle protein. Excess protein intake in the diet is converted to fat and not excreted.

Pathological Weight Control Among Athletes

Athletes who compete in sports that have a weight component or in which scores and appearance are contingent on success commonly have a team policy regarding body weight. This emphasis on appearance is one factor that could lead to disordered eating patterns that result in chronic physical and psychological medical conditions. Many athletes who find themselves in this kind of situation are at risk to drop out of athletic participation, either when the problem is identified and then treated, or when the athlete is forced to discontinue his career all together. The problem of disordered eating patterns can lead to disordered conditions known as anorexia nervosa, bulimia nervosa, and binge eating disorder. While these illnesses occur at a greater rate among females than among males, it is not unusual to find male athletes practicing these same kinds of disordered eating patterns.

Anorexia is characterized by an obsessive effort to lose weight or maintain a thin profile while on a diet. Anorexic athletes may eat, but the meal portions are restrictive. Anorexia is an obsessive disorder, in that the athlete feels as though he must be as thin as possible to be competitive. Bulimia is a condition in which an athlete may eat great quantities of food in one sitting (often called "binge eating") and then purge, typically by vomiting before the food has had a chance to leave the stomach on its way to being digested. It has been estimated that nearly half of all NCAA programs have reported athletes being treated for anorexia or bulimia in the past several years, with nearly 90 percent of those athletes being women. These conditions are more common and much more serious than was once thought. Very likely, a case of disordered eating is present in most athletic programs, from high school through elite-level Olympic and professional sport teams.

Disordered eating patterns lead to other more complicated medical and nutritional issues. The nutritional issues have been clearly defined in both anorexia and bulimia. Anorexic and bulimic athletes (either through the starvation practices of anorexia or the purging practices of bulimics) cannot get the nutrients they need to sustain a high level of physical performance. Athletes with anorexia simply do not get enough calories, because they do not eat. The pattern is a fast weight loss and increased muscle wasting (using the protein from the muscles as an energy source instead of carbohydrate and fat). The fat weight comes off first because it is the most readily available source of energy during a prolonged fast. Then, the protein must be used as the energy source, because few energy sources are left for the body to call upon in these conditions. Bulimic athletes face similar problems. Bulimics will eat, but then purge before any of the food can be digested and subsequently absorbed by the small intestine to be used

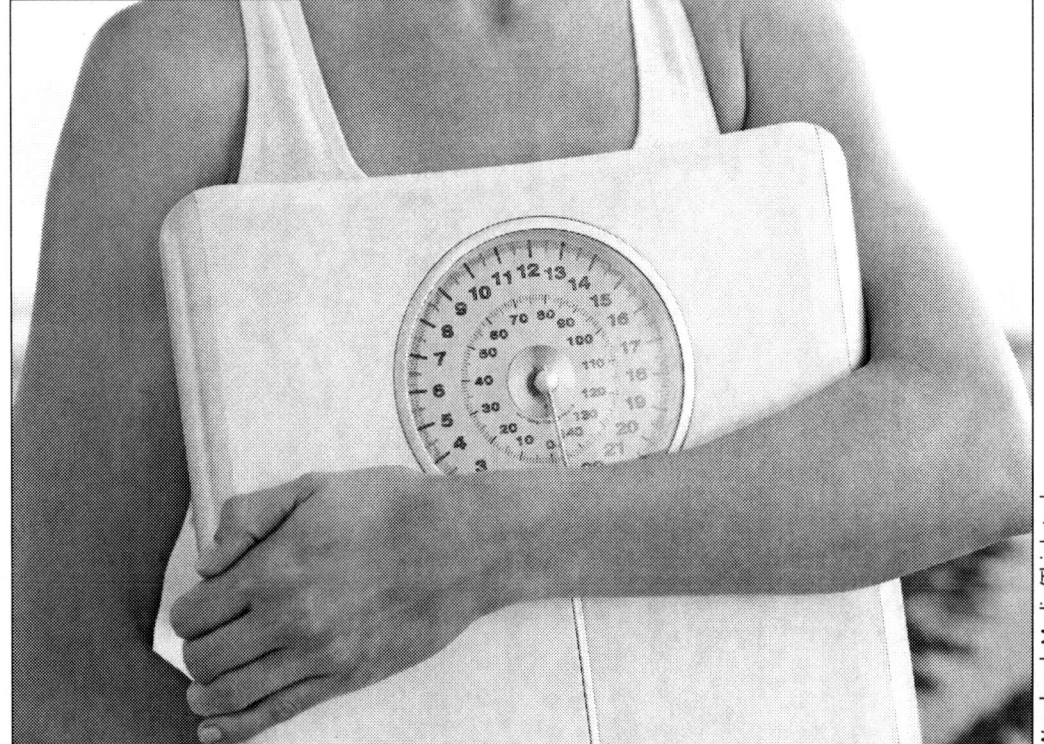

Disordered eating patterns lead to other more complicated medical and nutritional issues.

as energy. The chronic energy deficits experienced by both anorexic and bulimic athletes lead to a degradation in performance.

Along with the reduction in caloric consumption and chronic negative energy balance associated with these eating disorders, reductions in much-needed vitamins and minerals occur. A reduction in the essential vitamins leads to other medical issues, such as menstrual irregularities in female athletes. While it may be true that some athletes will experience secondary amenorrhea during a competitive season, this condition is usually associated with the high-intensity training experienced by the athlete. However, most of these athletes will return to a normal menstrual cycle after the competitive season has been completed. Patients with chronic eating disorders typically have a more persistent condition of amenorrhea.

Summary

The ability to stay in a constant energy balance has been shown to be very advantageous in both the prevention of injuries during practice and to the achievement of a successful athletic performance. Athletes who are in a negative energy balance, even for a short period of time, will exhibit decrements in performance. Athletes in a constant positive energy balance often experience the negative consequences of adding fat weight when the goal was to add lean (muscle) weight. Athletes should strive for an energy balance throughout the day by replacing the typical and culturally acceptable three-meals-a-day pattern in favor of small but frequent meals.

Section Five

Glossary

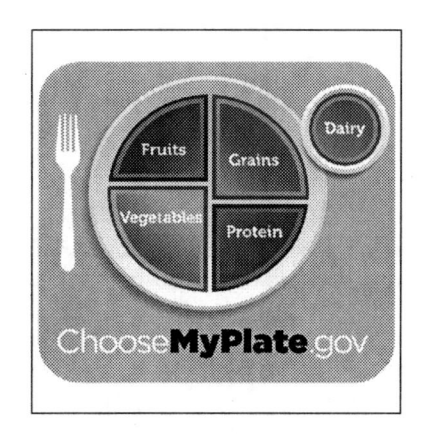

Adenosine Triphosphate (ATP): The form of energy the body uses at a cellular level.

Adequate Intake (AI): The amount of a nutrient believed to cover the needs of almost all individuals in the group. This designation implies that further research is needed and that this value is based on limited data.

Adipose Tissue Triglyceride: Triglyceride stored in the adipose tissue.

Aerobic Metabolism: Also known as oxidative phosphorylation. An energy system that generates ATP from the breakdown of carbohydrates, fats, or proteins. This system can supply ATP on a fairly limitless basis.

American Dietetic Association (ADA): A leading professional organization that governs the practice of nutrition and dietetics. A credible source for food and nutrition information (www.eatright.org).

Amino Acid: The smallest unit of a protein.

Anaerobic Glycolysis: An energy system that generates ATP fairly rapidly from the breakdown of glucose.

Anorexia Athletica: Not an official eating disorder listed in the DSM-IV, but is common in athletes who use energy restriction and/or excessive exercise to maintain a low body weight in an attempt to enhance performance.

Anorexia Nervosa: A medical condition characterized by an intense fear of becoming fat and a refusal to maintain a healthy body weight.

Antioxidant: Compound that protects cells from free radical damage.

Bioelectrical Impedance Analysis: A body-composition assessment technique that uses an electrical current to measure resistance and then estimate percent body fat.

Biological Value: Compares the amount of nitrogen absorbed from the food with that retained in the body for maintenance and growth.

Body Mass Index (BMI): A weight-for-height standard that is related to body-fat content.

Bulimia Nervosa: A medical condition characterized by consuming large quantities of food (binging) followed by a compensatory behavior to prevent body weight gain.

Carbohydrate Loading: A technique that begins about a week before an endurance event with the purpose of maximizing glycogen stores. It is characterized by a few days of glycogen depletion with exercise and low to moderate carbohydrate intake followed by glycogen repletion with tapered exercise and high carbohydrate intake.

Case Studies: Published observations on a person or group of people.

Chylomicron: A lipoprotein that transports dietary triglycerides.

Chyme: A mixture of partially digested food and stomach secretions.

Complete Protein: A protein that contains all nine essential amino acids.

Dietary Approaches to Stop Hypertension (DASH): Research-based guidelines showing that diets moderate in sodium and rich in fruits and vegetables that include low-fat dairy and lean protein may be effective in improving blood pressure (www.dashdiet.org).

Dietary Guidelines for Americans: Guidelines published by the USDA and the Department of Health and Human Services (www.health.gov/dietaryguidelines) that are designed to meet nutrient requirements, promote health, and prevent disease in people over the age of two.

Dietary Reference Intakes (DRIs): Developed by the Food and Nutrition Board of the Institute of Medicine in the United States and Health Canada. Umbrella term for nutrient recommendations. Includes Recommended Dietary Allowance (RDA), Adequate Intake (AI), Estimated Energy Requirement (EER), and Upper Level (UL).

Dietary Supplement Health and Education Act (DSHEA): Legally defined, a dietary supplement as a product (other than tobacco) added to the total diet that contains at least one of the following: a vitamin, mineral, amino acid, herb, botanical, or concentrate, metabolite, constituent, or extract of such ingredients or combination of any ingredient described previously.

Digestion: The process of mechanically and chemically breaking down larger consumed food molecules to smaller particles that can be absorbed across the wall of the small intestine.

Dipeptide: Two amino acids joined together.

Disaccharides: Two monosaccharides joined together (e.g., lactose, maltose, sucrose).

Diverticulosis: A medical condition characterized by pockets forming in the large intestine. These pockets generally come from years of pressure from straining to pass stool.

Dual Energy X-Ray Absorptiometry (DXA): A body-composition assessment technique that uses X-rays to measure bone density and percent body fat.

Dyslipidemia: A term to describe abnormal serum lipoproteins, especially elevated total cholesterol and LDL cholesterol, and lowered HDL cholesterol.

Eating Disorders Not Otherwise Specified (EDNOS): A category of eating disorders that describes individuals who do not meet all, but have some, of the specific criteria for anorexia nervosa or bulimia nervosa.

Electrolyte: A substance that separates into ions in solution and, therefore, conducts an electrical current; include sodium, chloride, and potassium.

Energy Balance: Energy (calories) consumed equals energy (calories) used or burned. Body weight is stable in this condition.

Energy Expenditure Due to Physical Activity (EEPA): Any movement of the body above rest, including purposeful exercise, representing 15 to 30 percent of the total daily energy expenditure in most individuals.

Energy Nutrients: Nutrients that provide calories (or energy) (e.g., carbohydrates, proteins, and fats).

Enriched Foods: Some of the nutrients lost with processing that are added back to the foods.

Epidemiological Studies: Studies that report associations or correlations between two variables, generally on larger populations.

Essential Amino Acid: Any of the nine amino acids that must be consumed in the diet because the body cannot synthesize them.

Estimated Energy Requirement (EER): Used to estimate the energy needs of an average person using gender, height, weight, age, and physical-activity level.

Euhydration: A state of adequate fluid balance.

Evidence-Based Medicine: The conscientious, explicit, and judicious use of current best evidence in making decisions about the care of individual patients.

Experimental Studies: Research studies or projects that use the scientific process or method to test a research question or hypothesis.

Fat-Free Mass: Tissue absent of all extractable fat. Often used interchangeably with lean body mass, although not technically equivalent.

Fat-Soluble Vitamins: Vitamins that dissolve in fat; Vitamins A, D, E, and K.

Fatty Acid: The simplest unit of a lipid; contains long chains of carbon molecules bound to each other and to hydrogen atoms.

Female Athlete Triad: Term is used to bring together three related conditions: disordered eating (usually a low energy intake), amenorrhea, and osteopenia or osteoporosis (low bone density).

Fiber: A chain of glucose molecules that the human body cannot break down (digest) due to lack of appropriate enzymes.

Food Label: A result of the Nutrition Labeling and Education Act of 1990. Displays nutrient content of a food product. Regulated by the United States Food and Drug Administration (FDA; www.fda.gov).

Fortified Foods: Foods that have added nutrients that may not naturally occur in the product.

Four-Compartment Body-Composition Model: Model that separates the body components into fat, muscle, bone, and water.

Gastrointestinal Reflux Disease (GERD): A medical condition where the acidic chyme from the stomach enters the esophagus.

Glucogenic Amino Acid: An amino acid that can be converted to glucose via gluconeogenesis.

Gluconeogenesis: A process of synthesizing glucose from non-carbohydrate precursors.

Glucose: The usable form of carbohydrate in the body.

Glycemic Index: A rating system used to describe a food's potential to raise blood glucose and insulin levels. The incremental area under the plasma glucose curve in response to 50 grams of available carbohydrate, in the fasted state, compared to a reference food (glucose or white bread).

Glycemic Load: The quantity of carbohydrate in food multiplied by the glycemic index of the food.

Glycogen: The storage form of carbohydrate in the human body; found in both the liver and in skeletal muscle.

Health Claims: Statements approved for use by the FDA that describe the relationship between a nutrient and a specific disease or health-related condition.

Hyperlipidemia: A term to describe elevated serum lipoproteins, especially total cholesterol and LDL cholesterol.

Hypohydration: A state of low levels of body water due to intake being less than loss; often called dehydration.

Hyponatremia: A general medical condition meaning low serum sodium. Exercise-associated hyponatremia is specific to athletes and usually occurs with long-duration endurance events.

Ideal/Desirable Body Weight: A body weight associated with the lowest risk of death; may not be practical for all individuals.

Incomplete Protein: A protein that lacks one or more essential amino acids.

Intramuscular Triglyceride: Triglyceride stored within the skeletal muscle.

Ketoacidosis: A medical condition characterized by excessive ketone levels in the blood, resulting in an acidic state and potential tissue damage.

Kilocalorie (kcal): The amount of heat required to raise the temperature of one kilogram of water by one degree Celsius. Common term used to describe energy content of food or energy expended.

Lacto-ovo-vegetarian: A person who consumes plants, dairy foods, and eggs.

Lacto-vegetarian: A person who consumes plants and dairy foods.

Lean Body Mass: Contains a small percentage of essential fat; generally refers to muscle (skeletal and smooth), bone, and water. Often used interchangeably with fat-free mass.

Lipoprotein: Vehicle that transports lipids through the lymph and circulatory systems. Contains a lipid center surrounded by a protein shell.

Macronutrients: Nutrients required in larger quantities, including carbohydrates, lipids, proteins, and water.

Megadose: Nutrient intake beyond those needed to prevent deficiency; at least 10 times the estimated requirement.

Meta-Analysis: Similar to a review article, except the authors take data from other primary research articles and statistically reanalyze it to put the results on a level playing field.

Metabolism: A sum of all the chemical reactions in the body.

Micronutrients: Nutrients required in small or trace amounts, including vitamins and minerals.

Monosaccharide: The simplest unit of a carbohydrate (e.g., glucose, fructose, and galactose).

Monounsaturated Fatty Acids: Fatty acids with double bonds between some of the carbons and, hence, room to add more hydrogen molecules. Monounsaturated fats have one double bond; common examples include olive oil and canola oil.

MyPlate: A Food Guidance System designed and supported by the United States Department of Agriculture (USDA; www.choosemyplate.gov).

National Weight Control Registry: Created in 1994, it is the largest research investigation of successful weight-loss maintenance, containing data on more than 5,000 individuals who have lost significant amounts of weight and who have maintained that weight loss for extended amounts of time (www.nwcr.ws).

Nitrogen Balance: A physiological state in which dietary nitrogen consumed equals nitrogen output. The classical method for determining dietary protein requirements.

Nutrient Content Claims: Claims approved by the FDA that define quantities of nutrients in a product.

Nutrition: The scientific study of the relationship between food and health and disease.

Office of Dietary Supplements: An office of the National Institutes of Health. A reliable source for information about dietary supplements (ods.od.nih.gov).

Omega-3 Fatty Acid: An essential fatty acid (it must be consumed in the diet). Found in fatty fish, flax seed, and certain nuts (e.g., walnuts and almonds).

Omega-6 Fatty Acid: An essential fatty acid (it must be consumed in the diet). Found in many vegetable oils.

Peer-Reviewed Journal Article: An article that has gone through a formal review process by other experts in the field. This process ensures that published research studies have been scrutinized by impartial experts for the soundness of the research methods utilized, and that the conclusions of the authors are supported by their research findings.

Phosphocreatine System: An energy system that produces ATP rapidly, but has a limited production capacity.

Phytochemicals: Biologically active compounds found in plants that may play a role in health promotion or the prevention of disease.

Plethysmography: A body-composition assessment technique that uses air displacement to measure body volume and then estimate percent body fat.

Polypeptide: Many amino acids joined together.

Polysaccharides: Long chains of monosaccharides (e.g., starch, fiber, and glycogen).

Polyunsaturated Fatty Acids: Fatty acids with double bonds between some of the carbons and, hence, room to add more hydrogen molecules. Polyunsaturated fatty acids have more than one double bond and are commonly found in many vegetable oils.

Primary Research Article: Published results of a research study or experiment.

Protein Digestibility-Corrected Amino Acid Score (PDCAAS): The USDA's official method for determining protein quality, accounting for both amino acid composition and digestibility.

PubMed: A database of biomedical articles from the National Library of Medicine database (www.pubmed.gov).

Recommended Dietary Allowance (RDA): Set to meet the needs of almost all (97 to 98 percent) individuals in the reference group.

Registered Dietitian: A legal credential governed by the Commission on Dietetic Registration of the American Dietetic Association. A specialized college degree, supervised practice experience, and passing of a national examination are required to earn the credential.

Resting Metabolic Rate (RMR): The amount of energy the body expends just to maintain itself at rest. It is largest component (60 to 75 percent) of the total daily energy expenditure. Also known as resting energy expenditure.

Review Article: A summary of previous studies that have been published up to that point in time.

Saturated Fatty Acids: Fatty acids where the carbon molecules are saturated with hydrogen. They tend to be solid at room temperature and are associated with an increased risk of developing hyperlipidemia when overconsumed.

Short-Term Fatigue: Occurs when exercise intensity rises to levels that disturb the body's ability to break down and transport the carbon, hydrogen, and oxygen molecules in macronutrients.

Skinfold Assessment: A body-composition assessment technique that uses a caliper to measure the thickness of subcutaneous body fat.

Sports Dietetics: The specific practice of using the Nutrition Care Process in counseling athletes and active individuals. These services are provided by a registered dietitian and/or a certified specialist in sports dietetics (CSSD).

Sport Drinks: A term usually used to describe a beverage containing carbohydrate and electrolytes.

Sports Nutrition: The scientific study of the relationship between food and nutrients and athletic performance.

Sports, Cardiovascular, and Wellness Nutrition (SCAN): A dietetics practice group of the American Dietetic Association composed of dietitians who practice in the areas of cardiovascular, sports, and wellness nutrition (www.scandpg.org).

Starch: The storage form of carbohydrate in plants; is abundant in the human diet.

Structure-Function Claims: These claims are not approved by the FDA. Products using these claims must include a disclaimer statement.

Thermic Effect of Food: The energy expended to digest and metabolize food, representing only 5 to 10 percent of the total daily energy expenditure.

Three-Compartment Body-Composition Model: Model that separates the body components into fat and lean body mass, with an independent assessment of body water.

Total Daily Energy Expenditure: Energy expended in a 24-hour period.

Trans Fatty Acids: Fatty acids with hydrogen molecules being on opposite sides of the double bonds. This solid vegetable-based compound has great cooking properties, but is associated with an increased risk of developing dyslipidemia when overconsumed.

Triglyceride: A form of lipid in the human diet and the form stored in the human body. A triglyceride contains three fatty acid molecules joined together by a three-carbon alcohol called glycerol.

Tripeptide: Three amino acids joined together.

Two-Compartment Body-Composition Model: Model that separates the body components into fat and lean body mass.

Underwater Weighing: A body-composition assessment technique that uses body density measurements to estimate percent body fat.

Upper Level (UL): The highest amount of a nutrient that when consumed regularly will unlikely result in adverse health effect.

Vegan: A person who consumes only plant foods.

Water-Soluble Vitamins: Vitamins that dissolve in water; includes the B vitamins and Vitamin C.

Weight Cycling: The process of continuously losing and gaining weight.

Wheat Flour: Any flour made from wheat; it may contain white flour, unbleached flour, or whole-wheat flour. May also contain fiber.

Whey Protein: The liquid portion of curdled milk that contains a high concentration of branched-chain amino acids (e.g., isoleucine, leucine, and valine).

White Flour: Flour that has been refined and bleached. Lacks significant fiber.

Whole-Grain Flour: A non-refined grain; only the husk is removed. Contains fiber.

About the Author

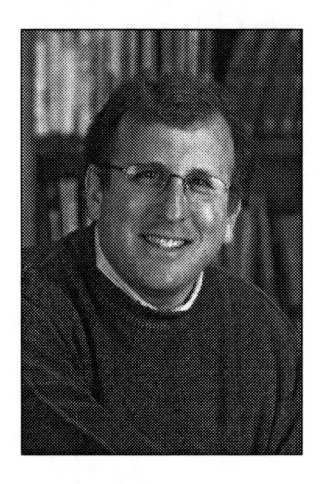

Jason Conviser, Ph.D., FACSM, is one of the leading experts in the fitness and wellness industry, both within the United States and throughout the world. He is best known for his insights and entrepreneurial work for clients' interests in sports medicine, metabolic syndrome, and bringing health care to the general public outside of a clinical environment. His work takes him throughout the United States, as well as China, Italy, Brazil, Indonesia, Israel, Columbia, Turkey, Mexico, and Australia. Dr. Conviser has conducted hundreds of health and wellness presentations to groups ranging in size from 20 to 3,000 and has been an invited speaker to 38 international conferences. He has co-authored five books, *INSIGHTs on Exercise: A Guide to Improving Your Health Through Fitness, Handbook of Acceleration Training, Exercise Testing and Program Design: A Fitness Professional's Handbook, Try Fitness First,* and *Osteogenic Loading: A New Modality to Facilitate Bone Density Development,* as well as authored numerous articles in scientific journals, trade publications, and large distribution newspapers. He was a past consultant and exercise physiologist to the Duchess of York, Sarah Ferguson.